FIBROMYALGIA SELF-HELP HANDBOOK

HOW TO MANAGE FIBROMYALGIA, HAVE LESS PAIN, MORE ENERGY, FEEL HAPPIER, LIKE A SUPERHERO ROCKSTAR!

WRITTEN BY SANDRA BELLAMY (AKA) ACE FIBRO GIRL

FIBROMYALGIA SELF-HELP HANDBOOK

How To Manage Fibromyalgia, Have Less Pain, More Energy, Feel Happier, Like A Superhero Rockstar!

Text And Illustration Copyright © 2019 Sandra Bellamy

Cover design by Sandra Bellamy

If you enjoy reading this book then please leave an honest review on Amazon.

DEDICATION

This book is dedicated to those who live day in day out with fibromyalgia; who love to challenge the norm; who like to think outside the box; who like to defy conventions; who always seek their own answers in life, and who like to break the rules and create their own rules to live by.

CONTENTS

"Be Your Own Superhero And Save Yourself From Pain!"

"Don't Let Your Limits Limit You!"

"Your Mind Is More Powerful Than Your Body – Make Sure You Exercise It Regularly."

"Live For You, Be Your Authentic Self And Live Your Life, Your Way."

PREFACE

This book is based on 10 observations

Observation no 1

There are thousands of people around the world who, like you, have fibromyalgia. Some go to a full-time job and lead a relatively 'normal life'. Some work part-time. Some can work some times and not at other times. Some are bed ridden for long periods at a time. Some are on crutches, while others are in a wheelchair. So it can be assumed that fibromyalgia affects people in different ways, but why?

Observation no 2

There are those with fibromyalgia, who right now feel that no one understands them. There are those that will publicly express how much pain they are in, how much medication they are on, and that you don't know how it feels, unless you are a 'sufferer'. Whilst there are those that keep quiet about it, and who 'suffer' in silence, or maybe not?

Observation no 3

Whilst all those with fibromyalgia have that one thing in common, it can be noted that they 'react' to it in different ways. But what is the significance of this?

Observation no 4

The pharmaceutical industry is worth big money, so it's in their financial interests for those with fibromyalgia to be given medication and the more the merrier for them.

Observation no 5

Those who are on medication sometimes report that it makes no difference.

Observation no 6

Medications can have serious side effects. Often you will need a pill, to counteract the effects of another, and this can be a never ending cycle of pill – effect – need another pill – effect – need another pill! Who is this benefitting?

Observation no 7

People with fibromyalgia are taught conventional ways to manage it. But do these really work? And what are the alternatives to getting a better quality of life?

Observation no 8

The world has changed. You are living in the information age with easy access to a wealth of knowledge about various health conditions and to people sharing ideas and experiences with each other. It is easier now, more than ever, to self-diagnose; to discover remedies you may previously have never known about; to find out answers that you may never have asked the question for, and to find things to help yourself. But will you help yourself? Will you be a sheep, or the shepherd leading your own way?

Observation no 9

There seems to be no definite conclusion that anyone is willing to say – That's why I have fibromyalgia, until this book...

Observation no 10

Two of the biggest problems fibromyalgia sufferers face is how to have less pain and more energy. But if there were methods, techniques, and things to decrease your pain and increase your energy, would you try them?

There is a lot of fear in the world, and of trying new things. There is something unsettling about getting out of your comfort zone, especially when in pain, but what is the alternative? You keep doing what you are doing, over and over again and you keep getting the same result. What is it you are afraid of? You have the condition anyway, things are not improving, but getting worse, and you feel like you are in a vicious cycle of pain. Do you want to break that cycle? Do you want to feel a breath of fresh air, to read of a different approach, however absurd it may seem to be? I mean, even if you learn just one new thing that could take a little of your pain away, wouldn't it be worth it? What have you got to lose by exploring new possibilities and ways of 'managing' this condition?

If you feel your current methods of managing fibromyalgia are simply not working, if you have an incredibly open mind to new possibilities, and you want effective ways to decrease your pain and have more energy, then please read on...

If any of these observations have resonated with you and if you haven't done so already, please invest in this book and I will reveal to you **how to manage fibromyalgia, have less pain, more energy, feel happier, like a superhero rockstar!**

But before we begin our journey together, I think there is something you should know....

PROLOGUE

"You are fitter than I am because you can walk into the city, whereas I have a bad back."

'Why is he telling me this, even before he examines me?'

This was the first doctor I saw and I would like to say that this experience got better, but it didn't. He concluded it was bad posture, even before he examined me! And the fact he had a nurse sat next to him, as soon as I walked through the door, made me feel uneasy.

Nothing changed after the examination. He concluded it was definitely posture. As you can imagine, I was neither happy with the way the appointment had been conducted or concluded. So I managed to find an outside body of the NHS to file a complaint for me, and after letters going back and forth, detailing the full extent of my examination complaint, and believe me, there was more than just this foul play, I was able to get another doctor to give me a second opinion.

This doctor did pressure point testing, as I expected from my research about tests for fibromyalgia, which said there is no blood test for it but x amount of pressure points that people with fibromyalgia experience pain from. As I almost always nearly pass out from blood tests, I was really relieved to know it was going to be this type of test, especially as I already knew pressure points that hurt on my arms, my neck and back. He concluded that I did have fibromyalgia and asked if I would like to be prescribed medication for the pain. I confirmed with the doctor that what he was offering me is used to treat depression, he said yes, but nerve damage too. I declined and told him I do not want any meds; I don't like taking meds if I can help it. That was in January 2012, and I got a letter confirming my official diagnosis of fibromyalgia, with a summary of my examination appointment and the fact I had declined the medication which he felt was for the best, as I manage myself and my condition well and that was my preference.

But how did I get to that point?

I first discovered something different about the way my feet felt back in 2010, when I was managing a two-floor outdoor camping and leisure shop.

In 2011, I was working in a well-known brand of electrical store, selling TVs, computers, audio equipment and accessories. It hurt to carry a 21" or 19" LED TV from the stockroom to the shop floor for the customer to take away, and even carrying a tray of teas for the staff would cause my arms to go into spasms. It took up to 40 minutes for the Ibuprofen to start working and numb the pain so I could get back to work. It worried me that I had to go off the shop floor in pain, that the job I wanted to keep, was causing the situation that made me in pain.

The succession of events is a bit blurry in regards to timescale, but I do remember being referred to a podiatrist for a 'foot problem' that caused swelling and made it hard for me to walk. The consultation with him, led to some new insoles being especially made for me. Did they work? What do you think? Exactly – nope! What I can reveal to you right now, which does work, and has worked for me for years, is trainer socks with ventilation panels – WORN THROUGHOUT THE WHOLE YEAR, including all the winter months!! Did I tell you this book is about getting out of your comfort zone? If something works, give it a go! I get my trainer socks from Tesco, (and no, I am not endorsing Tesco – I am just saying!), they are inexpensive for a multi-pack, and are smart black ones, making them suitable for work. The most important thing that prevents my feet swelling is the ventilation panels in them for breathability. Not all trainer socks have these ventilation panels, and that is why your feet will continue to swell if you don't get trainer socks with ventilation panels in them. So please listen to me if you have feet swelling and do as I do. No more 'normal' socks, or 'normal length' socks; are worn by me in the day. At night if I am not wearing trainer socks, I sometimes wear slipper socks, and I wear memory foam slippers at home all the time, with my trainer socks, which are far more supportive than normal slippers and the cushioning helps to prevent feet swelling and pain. If you have 'normal' slippers, go and get yourself some memory foam slippers today, not other foam, it has to be memory foam, take a week to get used to them with your trainer socks with ventilation panels and watch your feet as they should appear to be less red and have reduced swelling. If you see an improvement, do this consistently for months, and if it works then DON'T go back to normal socks or normal slippers EVER again. If you do revert back to your old habits, after a few days, you will likely notice you have the problem back again.

Both of my feet had a tendency to swell so badly, that by 2012, the year of my fibromyalgia diagnosis, I could barely walk from my self-contained studio flat bedroom to the toilet, and that happened on more than one occasion. At that time I was looking for work, but how could I work for any company, when my feet would not even allow me to walk from one room to the other and I nearly ended up crawling along the floor? I had to hold onto furniture just to make the journey, and try not to put the full weight of my feet directly on the floor. I can recall the redness and swelling on the sides of my feet spreading underneath them. Thank goodness I worked out that trainer socks are the answer to my prayers. That was the first new habit I formed, to change my life and stop 'suffering' like I had been. Most people would stop doing that in winter, 'oh, it's too cold for that' they would think to themselves, and so they may revert back to their old ways. To those I say, do you want to improve your quality of life or not? Make no excuses and wear these ALL year round, even in the harshest of weathers. Try two pairs if you must, but any sign of swelling and you must revert back to one pair. I can't say they are definitely going to work for you, but you have nothing to lose by trying them out. Do you want to do things that may seem a bit illogical under certain circumstances to change your life and experience less pain? It's your choice! Isn't it empowering to know that you have a choice, even as a fibro 'sufferer' – you can choose to suffer less!! Putting you in control and in the driving seat of your own life.

What happened after the podiatrist and before my diagnosis in January 2012?

Good question. I remember being sent to a physiotherapist, he said my outer arm muscles were strong, but my inner arm muscles are weak. After he asked me to do some homework – exercises at home, and I was in so much pain, he concluded that as they were simple Pilates and yoga exercises, they should not cause me that much pain, and there was something wrong that needed further investigation. So I got referred to see a hip specialist.

When seeing the hip specialist, I revealed that I could still feel the exact pain of my accidents I had in 1996, from certain pressure points on both arms, when I tore the tendon in my right arm and damaged the ligaments a week and a half later in my left arm, due to me putting all the pressure on it because I was no longer actively using the right. I remember my ex had to cut up food for me when I could not use my right arm. The hip specialist concluded that my hip was slightly out of alignment from where it should be, but he would not have noticed it, had he not been specifically asked to look at it. This came as no surprise to me because my mum told me I was born with a clicky hip. But what I was surprised about, he mentioned a word I had never heard of before in my life – fibromyalgia! "I am not saying you have it". And that was about it. No explanation for why he had said that word to me, and in such a random, casual fashion, it felt weird. Of course the mystery over this word, in association with my examination, left me with the compelling urge of curiosity to Google the term 'fibromyalgia' and see what comes up!

Later, I Googled, 'my legs feel like they have been run over by a bus' and fibromyalgia came up, so now I knew that the word fibromyalgia and the pain I felt in my body are related, it was time I paid a visit to the doctor to see if I had it and you know the rest.

PART 1
PREPARE TO BE A
SUPERHERO ROCKSTAR!

CHAPTER 1
HOW TO MANAGE FIBROMYALGIA, HAVE LESS PAIN, MORE ENERGY, FEEL HAPPIER, LIKE A SUPERHERO ROCKSTAR!

INTRODUCTION

This is no ordinary fibromyalgia book; it's unlike any other book you will have ever read before. This book does not tell you to take CBD oil, it's not discussing which pharmaceutical medications to take and it's not talking about patches to buy. This revolutionary Fibromyalgia Self-Help Handbook shows you a truly remarkable and unique "Superhero Rockstar" holistic way to manage your fibromyalgia, to enable you to have less pain, more energy and feel happier, and I am living proof it really works! This book takes you by the hand, step-by-step, and explains exactly how to decrease your pain in 25 aspects of your life, so you can live a happier, healthier, more energetic and fulfilling life, in spite of your fibromyalgia. By being more informed about what's most effective for coping with your fibromyalgia in multiple aspects of your life, you'll get your fibro working for you, rather than against you, through implementing positive action steps, which will dramatically improve the quality of your life. You will literally be given the antidotes to your pain to stop you from suffering like you have been.

WHO IS THIS BOOK FOR?

This book is for those with fibromyalgia, those who think they show signs of having fibromyalgia; for family, friends, or loved ones of those who have the condition, and for anyone and every-one who is keen and eager to know more about fibromyalgia and how to manage it to have less pain, more energy and feel happier. If you feel like fibromyalgia is ruining your life and taking over it, if you feel like you are going insane not knowing what to do for the best and you are desperate to get practical, helpful advice, that is actionable, direct and to the point, so you can finally take back control of your life; have more happiness; more energy and more freedom from your pain, then this is definitely the book for you.

I truly believe that having fibromyalgia saved my life, because be-fore that I was depressed for years and throughout my childhood. I had suicidal thoughts, and after 6 months of taking time to come to terms with having a disability for life, in an instant I stopped hav-ing that negative mindset that had plagued me for years and intui-tively knew I had to stop it or it would make my fibro pain much worse! They say it takes a significant life-changing event to truly change your life and jolt it like a lightening bolt; well this is exactly what happened to me. I went from thoughts about dying and death, with negativity frequently on my mind, to being joyful, hap-py, younger, and more vibrant and energetic than ever before, with the help of another major event that year which I will share with you in chapter 2. I know you must be wondering how on earth can this be possible? But believe me it is. In this handbook, I reveal precisely what you need to do, to have the most incredible, extraordinary and superpower charged fibro live ever! So you will no longer be confused about what course of action to take to re-duce your pain and stop your fibro from flaring up.

In the chapters that follow, I will give you unique insight into how I manage this condition to reduce my pain, with insider secrets how to not just survive with fibro, but to truly flourish, thrive, and come alive, within it. I explain exactly how I am able to have, maintain and sustain, my energy levels, so you can do the same, with practical actionable steps you can implement immediately to get results rapidly. I will show you exactly how I can live a far happier life with my fibro than many others do, and how I just generally 'seem' to have a lot less pain! You will learn to zap depression where it hurts and how to stop it from returning. You will learn how control your anxiety and worry less and how to master your fibro, so you are always in control of it, not the other way around. You will learn what foods to eat and not to eat to reduce your pain, including one food you can find in your local supermarket to stop that 'my legs feel like they have been run over by a bus feeling'; what footwear to buy to stop your feet from swelling most of the time; what bed to get to ease your pain; what mindset to implement so you can unleash your fibro superpowers and make fibro work for you, instead of against you! I show you how you can do all these things and so much more, in this book. And just like fibromyalgia has changed my life for the better forever, I want this book to do the same for you.

WHO IS THIS BOOK NOT FOR?

If you are looking for a book that makes lots of references to sources of research and scientific notes, this is NOT the book for you. If you are looking to cure your fibro that is not what this book does. Rather it encourages you to learn how to manage your fibromyalgia effectively so that it doesn't destroy your quality of life. It gives you a revolutionary new way of thinking and seeing your fibromyalgia in a completely different light, so you can reduce your pain, get your energy back, live a happy life, and have fun in the process, despite your fibromyalgia.

So if you value your quality of life, if you are sick and tired of feeling sick and tired, with living in agony, pain and misery, with little energy and hope for the future, and it's making you feel depressed, if you have decided you can no longer go on like this and you need practical, helpful advice, you can put into action instantly to start making dramatic changes in your fibro life, to feel better, forever, this book IS DEFINITELY FOR YOU, so read on!

18 BENEFITS OF READING THIS BOOK!

Within these pages that follow, I will specifically reveal to you:

1) What fibromyalgia is and the cause of it.

2) The superpowers fibromyalgia gives you!

3) How to decrease your pain.

4) How to increase your energy.

5) How to get better quality sleep.

6) How to get a better quality of life.

7) How to overcome depression.

8) How to be happier.

9) How to have more confidence.

10) How to decrease your anxiety, worry less, and break through your fears.

11) What foods to cut out and add to your diet to have less pain and improve your wellbeing.

12) How to use the power of your mind to block out the pain and improve your life.

13) How to have a rockstar attitude that ensures you have fun and don't waste a moment of your precious life.

14) How to nourish your soul using my embrace your quirky philosophy to increase your self-love and personal power.

15) How to cope in everyday life situations and those with special meaning.

16) How to deal with your relationships with others, to keep pain at bay and goodness in your life. This includes your relationship with yourself, parents, family, partner and others.

You'll also discover:

17) My best-kept secret that even those closest to me didn't know about until they read this book!

18) How I do all the 'wrong' things to get the right results.

In this book I will explore these 25 aspects of your life that affect your fibro pain and how to reduce your pain within each of these areas:

1) Body.

2) Mind and mindset.

3) Foods you eat.

4) Medications you take.

5) Shopping.

6) Housework.

7) Clothes.

8) Attitude.

9) Thoughts.

10) Feelings.

11) Emotions.

12) Spirit/soul.

13) Intuition.

14) Mission, goals, ambitions and dreams.

15) Career/job

16) Lifestyle.

17) Weather.

18) Sleep.

19) Environment.

20) Hobbies.

21) Finances.

22) Friends and Family.

23) Relationship with yourself.

24) Relationship with others.

25) Love, intimacy and sex.

By the time you have finished reading this book, you will have all the antidotes, tools and techniques, to reduce your fibro pain, increase your energy levels and be happier, in spite of your fibromyalgia. If you follow EVERYTHING I teach you in this book, you will be a much more energetic version of yourself, you will know exactly what to do to keep your fibro pain

from flaring up in each aspect of your life, you will be more confident, less anxious, and feel so much better as a result. It's time to change your life, take charge and own your fibro, so that it never rules your life ever again.

ABOUT THIS BOOK

This book is part of the QUIRKY BOOKS range, and like many other Quirky Books, it crosses over genres. It is an AUTOBIOGRAPHICAL, SELF-HELP, HOW-TO BOOK. It is NOT a scientific account; it is a book based on my own experiences; what I have found out through my own research over the years; and the results I have achieved. My mission is to inspire and help people, just like you, to live a more vibrant energetic, happy and fulfilling life, in spite of your fibromyalgia.

WHAT CAN YOU EXPECT FROM THIS BOOK?

What you can expect to read is my personal fibro journey, what has worked for me and helped me to manage my condition well, to have less pain, and a better quality of life! I realise that some of my methods can be a bit far out and crazy – but big hint!! Sometimes crazy is what it takes to help yourself to live a better quality of life!!

A lot of people with fibro lack energy, are in constant conscious pain, sleep and rest a lot, don't do much that is physically demanding such as go clubbing until the early hours or to theme parks like I like to do, and a lot can't work full-time with it or at all. I have a ton of energy even on 3-4 hours sleep and I am naturally a hyper person and have not let my fibro stop that. In fact, now I lead my life, my way, because of my fibro, I am able to really bring out that energetic person in me, especially using the techniques I am about to show you in this book! Many people with fibro have sensitivity to noise and light; I love noise, lights, camera and action. Until I was made redundant, I worked in a full-time employed 'day job' for almost 5 years, and in the evenings I came home and worked on my own business stuff. I get bored easily and like to be doing stuff all the time, and this includes if I go away for the week. I am not a sunbather and rest type of person, but a doer and action taker, and I love to live life to the max. I am proudly an insomniac and use unconventional methods to get that deep sleep that most people with fibro can't achieve and I will divulge how to do that, in this book. I believe life should be one big party from beginning to end and that you can achieve the seemingly unachievable and live a happy and vibrant life; that you can live your dreams, even with fibro. I don't let my fibro own me and neither should you. But how do I do this? All will be revealed in this book!!

Throughout this book you with see both the word fibromyalgia and fibro (short for fibromyalgia), used interchangeably to mean the same thing – however, you will discover later on in this book, why I personally like to use the word fibro most of the time instead of the former, and how it can help if you do this too.

HOW TO USE THIS BOOK

This book should be read from cover to cover, all exercises completed within it, and every action taken, to give yourself the best possible chance of changing your life to decrease your conscious fibro pain, increase your energy levels, and make you feel happier overall.

Each section and chapter of this book should be completed in order, however, this book has also been designed so that after giving it a complete and thorough read through, you can also re-read each part or chapter on its own and still benefit from it and make improvements to your fibro life. For that reason, inevitably there are some crossovers and repetition between chapters and parts of this book. This is done with purpose and intent to show you how everything works together to reduce your pain, give you more energy, and make you feel happier as a result. Look at this book as a complete system for ensuring you have less pain, more energy, and feel happier, and each chapter and part of it being a building block to doing that. The more blocks you build, the stronger your foundation for getting, maintaining and sustaining, the most pain free, energetic, and happy fibro life as possible for you.

I have also included "key points to remember" throughout this book, to serve as a reminder of what you have learnt in a given chapter and to use for quick reference in the future after you have read through this whole book and want to remind yourself of the essentials of how to have less pain, more energy, and feel happier. If you are a skim reader, which I highly recommend you don't do with this book, the key points will cover the essential areas of your life that you must take control of and do the things I explain, if you want to make any improvement in your life. If you are one of those people who likes to skip to the back of the book first, which again, I highly recommend you don't, there is a summary of some of the main components of this book to get you started or to conclude with, how to reduce your pain, increase your energy, and feel happier, in spite of your fibro.

Just remember, if you don't take any action on anything I explain and show you in this book, don't expect to see any improvement. Changing your life takes work. The more action you take, the greater your chance of completely changing your life for the better, forever. You are the master of your life, no one else, so it's up to you to be disciplined enough to take action, follow through, and keep yourself on track, like the superhero rockstar, you were always born to be. Be your own superhero and save yourself from pain, unhappiness and lack of energy! You can do it, I believe in you.

WHAT IS FIBROMYALGIA AND WHAT ARE THE SYMPTOMS OF IT?

To put it in my own simple terms, fibromyalgia is a chronic pain condition that affects the nerves and muscles of the body. It is also known to be an autoimmune disease and although it is said you cannot die from fibromyalgia, you could get other life-threatening conditions because of it lowering your immune system.

To quote Wikipedia:

*"**Fibromyalgia (FM)** is a medical condition characterised by chronic widespread pain and a heightened pain response to pressure. Other symptoms include tiredness to a degree that normal activities are affected; sleep problems, and troubles with memory. Some people also report restless legs syndrome, bowel or bladder problems, numbness and tingling, and sensitivity to noise, lights or temperature. Fibromyalgia is frequently associated with depression, anxiety, and posttraumatic stress disorder. Other types of chronic pain are also frequently present."*

WHAT CAUSES FIBROMYALGIA?

To quote Wikipedia:

"The cause of fibromyalgia is unknown; however, it is believed to involve a combination of genetic and environmental factors with

half the risk attributed to each. The condition runs in families and many genes are believed to be involved. Environmental factors may include psychological stress, trauma, and certain infections. The pain appears to result from processes in the central nervous system *and the condition is referred to as a "central sensitization syndrome". Fibromyalgia is recognized as a disorder by the US National Institutes of Health and the American College of Rheumatology. There is no specific diagnostic test. Diagnosis involves first ruling out other potential causes and verifying that a set number of symptoms are present."*

There is no doubt in my own mind as to why I have fibromyalgia and to why many others have it too. From the research I have done, the people I speak to online about fibromyalgia; the groups I am in; and the forums I read, to sum up what causes fibromyalgia, in a word, it is trauma. Such as giving birth, accidents and abuse – which can be physical, sexual, mental, emotional, or a combination of any or all of them. I have never given birth and personally have never wished to, but I was the result of a forceps birth. I have had multiple accidents, including being knocked over by a moped 3 days before my 12th birthday, taking lessons on how to drive a moped and coming off it and going under the front wheel of a parked car – I stopped my lessons after that, and falling head first down 11 stone steps at work. I have had all of those other types of traumas too. So it is easy for me to see why I have this and I take responsibility and ownership for having been in those situations, even though I do not blame myself for the abuse and I know I did the best I could do in those situations at that time, as that former version of me. And this is absolutely key to managing fibromyalgia, to take ultimate responsibility and ownership of it. Something human beings like to do naturally, is to blame others for their condition or to adopt a victim attitude and mindset, because naturally, we do not want to think we are responsible for causing our own pain, but if we don't take responsibility for managing it, the pain will become unbearable. And whilst we don't have to accept we directly caused this to ourselves, we have to understand that we all have choices in life, even if we were weak at the time, even if we did not know what we were doing, or we felt powerless and trapped. Because by taking responsibility for the acknowledgment that we were in that situation in the first place, for whatever reason, we can begin to feel back in control and take back some of our personal power that may have been stolen from us recently or a long time ago. If we blame others, our power is with those we blame. We need all of our strength to accept we have this condition, for us to move forward and to be able to manage it in the best way possible for our self. We need to own our fibro so it doesn't own us, or our life. I like to believe everything happens for a reason and the why will uncover itself if we think about it and seek it, and if we can see the positive in every situation. Take Nick Vijucic the guy from YouTube known for "No Arms. No Legs. NO LIMITS". He may not have fibromyalgia, but he was born with no legs and no arms, yet he has a wife and kids and is an international world class speaker, inspiring everyone around the globe with his message that no matter what happens in life, you are born for a special purpose and never give up, if you get knocked down, then pick yourself up again and keep trying. I saw Nick at the 2015 National Achievers Congress in London and he was amazing. He proudly sat upright, in front of the audience, a torso with a flipper foot, a handsome face and a smile. He allowed himself to fall over and showed how he could get back up again by himself. He could have stayed all his life wallowing in self-pity; he could have looked at his disability as just that, and allowed himself to be and feel powerless, but he didn't. Neither does he deny that which is a part of him. He acknowledges it, adapts his life and lifestyle to it, and uses it to his advantage. He owns his power, he owns his energy, he owns his life, and he owns his disability and he honours it. We must do the same with our fibromyalgia. I want you to repeat these two power declarations right now: "I OWN MY FIBRO; IT DOES NOT OWN ME. I AM IN CONTROL; I FEEL MY POWER AND MY ENERGY." And these should be part of your daily morning affirmation routine from now onwards.

If this is the first time you have come across 'affirmations' and wonder what I am talking about, affirmations are short, powerful statements, that can change your thinking and your life. To affirm, means to confirm something is true. Affirmations are statements; that you use to say what you want to be true, as if it were already in existence and true. Therefore changing your thought patterns, your mental environment, and your own reality. Many of our thoughts are subconscious, and sadly, many of them are negative. We may say things to ourselves like, I feel in pain; I feel sick; I hurt; I don't want to get out of bed today; I hate life. If we keep saying these negative things over and over again to ourselves in our mind, how do you think we are going to feel? Notice the 'think', 'feel' correlation? What we think about, we manifest into a feeling. And if we feel bad, we focus on the thought of that feeling, making us feel more of that, it's a vicious cycle. What we focus on expands, and therefore we need to focus less on our pain and more on what makes us joyful, happy, and feel great. We need to counteract our negativity with positivity, by saying positive statements to ourselves, to change our beliefs, mindset and attitudes towards life, on a consistent daily basis, so we can then manifest those positive power statements into our conscious reality. If done consistently they work for me; they change my mood to be more positive; they change my thoughts to ones of optimism, giving me hope, instilling belief in myself; my own abilities, and capabilities, so they can work for you too. Think about having a set of silver metal scales in front of you, on the one side you have a heaped tablespoon of negativity and the other side you have a <u>tea</u>spoon of positivity, which one is winning? Which one is weighing down the other? Even writing this book to help you is super hard for me, because as I talk to you about my fibromyalgia, I am focusing more on the pain that comes with it, bringing up negative thoughts, feelings and emotions, to my conscious mind, when usually I would choose not to think about it and focus on seeing only the benefits, and mention it casually in conversation only when necessary. I have a morning routine of affirmations that I say to myself each day; that never includes the word fibro, but they include "I AM IN CONTROL. I FEEL MY POWER AND MY ENERGY." So if leaving the word FIBRO out completely would work better for you, then leave it out, adapt affirmations to what you want them to be for you – but always remember they need to be positive and said in present tense. The more you say positive statements to yourself, every morning, ideally in the mirror out loud as they tend to sink into the subconscious more; about what you want to feel, think, and believe, the more likely they are to come true. In effect, you are re-wiring your negative subconscious to become a positive consciousness, which can only be a good thing.

So why should trauma cause fibromyalgia? How does that work?

In a dangerous situation, such as abuse, where there is a threat, the body's natural response is 'fight or flight'. Meaning, you either want to run away from the situation, take flight and flee it, or stay there and fight it. Although fighting it may be literal, you may also keep quiet to stay safe, or do stuff you don't want to do, just to survive that situation – I call that damage limitation. But all the while you are considering what to do, which could be in a split second of time, your body is in this fight or flight mode, releasing chemicals such as adrenaline and cortisol. If you research the effects of these chemicals, it is noted, they can be okay in small dos-es, but prolonged exposure to them, can cause serious damage to your body, and I believe this is why people get fibromyalgia. I know from personal experience, in a past eight and a half year relationship, in the company of an abuser, that your body can be in constant flight or flight mode whilst you are in their presence, as you never know what will happen next, whether they will be nice to you, or grab hold of you, or shout at you. It is no wonder that your body becomes super sensitive to pain. It needs to be able to protect itself, because without feeling pain, you cannot know a situation is wrong and that is even more dangerous than the situation in and of itself.

BEFORE WE BEGIN

Before we begin, please bear in mind I am not offering medical advice, I am not a medical practitioner or health worker. I am not a therapist or counsellor. I am not a doctor and I am not saying anything or everything in this book will work for you. I am not advising or telling you to do anything, I am explaining what works for me and why, so you can see there is another way of managing fibromyalgia, an unconventional way, that some critics may even call irresponsible, yet is the most responsible way, because you are in control; you are in the driving seat; you are breaking free of the reins and claims that have enslaved you for years; you are coming into your own. You are no longer allowing fibro to dictate your life, it may be a part of you, but it is not who you are; your fibro does not define you, you do. Now is the time to free yourself from conditioned thinking; now is the time to be you!

First... a word of warning, what you are about to read may go against everything you are led to believe and told to do. I should let you know now that I am an individualist who plays by her own rules of life, that I am not dictated to by anything or anyone, and that I don't do normal and nor do I ever intend to, and this my friend, is how you manage fibromyalgia like a rockstar! So are you with me? Are you going to give me a high five? Let's do this and begin the fibro journey of your life! Here we go...

CHAPTER 2
PAIN INTO GAIN

As I mentioned before, it took me 6 months to come to terms with the fact that I have a disability for life. In July 2012, I made a conscious decision to choose to see the positives about fibromyalgia and the benefits it brought me. I thought I have this condition for life and I can either continue to think negatively about it which is not going to help me or make my condition any better, or I can choose to see the positives about it. I chose to have a positive mindset. Upon discovering that many people were bed ridden for hours by fibro (nickname for fibromyalgia), some were on crutches or in a wheelchair, I felt very lucky. I was taking no medications, and as far as I knew all other fibro sufferers were. I was abled bodied in so much as I could carry out my daily activities and work. And I am naturally a hyper and bubbly person, while most with fibro lack energy. I also knew, in that moment, I had to change my life for the better forever, and live my life for me. I wanted to make sure I have no regrets, and that should I have to be on crutches or in a wheelchair, later on in my life, that I had done everything within my power, to live life to the max, while I am able to. My mindset instantly shifted to be more positive! And thus, the concept of how to manage fibromyalgia like a rockstar, was born. But what about the superhero bit I hear you say, that comes in later...

First, I think there is something else you should know. It was also in 2012, the year of my fibromyalgia diagnosis, that my life changed completely for the better forever in another MAJOR way.

It was that year I started attending business seminars and entered into the world of personal and professional development, learning from some of the most influential life and business coaches, thought-leaders, entrepreneurs and specialists in their field. It was that year, I first saw Tony Robbins, known as the nation's #1 life and business strategist. Although he was talking to the masses in the room, he really made a huge impression on me. I felt like he was almost talking directly to me. He taught me how to change my state through the use of movement and music. So that every time I was in a state of feeling negative or lacking in energy, I could use movement and music to change that, and instantly become more happier and energised as a result. If you have ever seen Tony live, you will know that he is constantly getting the audience to stand up and jump up and down to music, and go around hugging people you don't know that are in the room with you. When I first got directed by him to go and hug strangers, this really got me out of my comfort zone. Up until that point, I did not like hugging anyone, or having any close physical contact, other than a boyfriend – if I had one, I was single at that time. Other than that, I would hug my parents to say goodbye, but that was it. I remember at this seminar, hugging a really large guy, both in height and body weight, who was predominantly bald on top, with some white flyaway hair. I thought if I can hug this guy, who was not attractive to me, then I could hug anyone. It still took me a while to get used to hugging, but now I do it naturally as part of my personality and I feel better for it. Now I am more open to people and lead a much more fulfilling life, and yes, as a fibro person hugs can hurt if people get on the wrong pressure points, but do you know what? If I am having such a great time, a lot of my conscious fibro pain just disappears, and I forget about it for some time. In 2016, I saw Tony Robbins again. I had been in quite a bit of pain before I got to this seminar with my neck, but once there, I allowed myself to think, 'it's fine, you will be okay, just jump up and down and have a great time', I did, and my neck pain healed quicker. In fact I jumped into people's arms and was still okay. One guy even lifted me up and I think I had my legs around him at some point, he was not bad looking so that is okay, but there was one older guy who loved hugging me just a little longer than was comfortable for me. The point is, do not let your limits, limit you. You become what you think about. In the seminar, I stopped thinking about my neck pain and let go of the fear that it would get worse, I told myself a positive affirmation and it worked. Positive self-talk, is absolutely crucial for being in less fibro pain and improving your wellbeing. It has to be a daily practice and habit, to form the mindset you need to not just survive but thrive as someone who has fibro. You have to be in control of your mind and your thoughts so they don't control you. You have to think positively or you will experience body pain as a result. Because of Fibromyalgia and this new found revelation of mind and body pain correlation, as well as this life changing seminar, where I noticed all of the skills, knowledge and experience I had that I could share and offer to the world, I finally felt I was worth something in life and that I mattered, that my life had purpose and meaning, my self-esteem increased and I started to truly love myself. I freed myself from depression that I had for years of my life since childhood, without medication, for life. And I owe that to my fibro, because without being diagnosed with fibro, I would not have swapped a negative mindset for a positive one and may never have gone to that seminar which changed my state and left a long-lasting legacy of self-love, self-worth, self-esteem, and the ability to know I can achieve anything in life that I set my mind to.

I've also seen Motivational Speaker, Author and Trainer Brendon Burchard live, and taken a course and some of his trainings. Among his teachings, I learnt it takes 21 days to form a new habit. So I created a new morning routine checklist and it works. We all have bad habits that are hard to break. We all have better habits we could adopt. The danger is not that we have habits, but that we have habits that do not serve us and get the best out of our lives. It may be in your own life, that you have adopted conventional habits for managing your fibromyalgia that are not really working for you; you don't understand why and you are trying your best, but nothing seems to be working and you feel like you are bashing your head against a brick wall in a pool of frustration. Or maybe you are new to fibromyalgia, and have no idea how to manage it to get the best results. So as you go through this book know that to truly change your life, you need to keep an open mind and try new things, but that it will take at least 21 days to form a new habit to get these things working and you pledge right here and now, to give it a go, that is all I ask of you. I cannot promise you they will work as everyone's fibromyalgia condition is unique to them, but all I can say, is if I can help you in any way, to have a little less conscious pain and a little better quality of life, then it will be worth it. So if you want to change your life and you want to know how to manage fibromyalgia like a superhero rockstar, read on!

CHAPTER 3
ROCKSTAR POWER

Let's examine the qualities of a rockstar.

Resilient

Open-minded

Creative

Kicking-butt

Strong

True to themselves

Action takers

Remarkable

What are the qualities of a rockstar performer?

- You lead by example, and are a leader in and of, your own life!

- You are not easily influenced, but you influence others through your commitment to your mission and your inspiration that nothing will stop you living your life, your way.

- You are passionate about life, act young, vibrant and energetic, and do not care what others think of you and your behaviour.

- You are your true authentic self, following your own path and standing out from the crowd.

- You play by your own rules in the game of life.

- You have the right can-do attitude and a relentless work ethic.

- Nothing fazes you.

- You are determined to not let anything stop you from achieving your goals, ambitions and dreams, and will adapt in whatever ways necessary to get them.

- You are a problem solver, a go-getter and an action taker.

- You will overcome obstacles and struggles to perform to the best of your ability.

- In fact, you see obstacles as challenges and will adapt to tackle those challenges head on to overcome them.

- You will change your direction in life if need be, and not allow fear of the unknown to consume you.

- You believe in yourself and your abilities, you know you have an inner strength and will get through anything life throws at you.

- You will work day and night to perfect your craft and are not afraid to stay up throughout the night to get stuff done, or just to enjoy life.

- You are a creative night owl.

- You know when to take some time off to recuperate and recharge, ready for your next energy burst, but you are not scared of being awake for hours to pursue your dreams and live in the night.

- You use music to sooth your soul and to elevate your state to one of energy.

- You manage your time well, are organised, and pack as much into your life as possible.
- You are positive, upbeat, and self-motivated to get the best out of life.
- You know your weaknesses and you are not perfect, but you don't dwell on negatives, instead, you focus on having a good time in life and playing to your strengths.
- You accept what is, but have hope and vision for the future, and make decisions that will endeavour to make your vision a reality by taking consistent action.

These are the rockstar qualities you need to have in order to give you the greatest possible chance of having the best quality of life as someone who has fibromyalgia. In essence, you have to almost forget you have fibro, and focus on those qualities of personality, attitude, and mindset, that will help you to decrease your pain and increase your pleasure, and therefore feel good factor and wellbeing. Believe me when I say, your fibro gives you superpowers and it is your superpower, you just don't realise it yet. But as we go through this fibro journey together, as you work your way through this book, you will be able to see just what is possible, and you will be able to master all 25 aspects of your life, to decrease your pain, increase your energy and feel happier, and not just read about these rockstar qualities, but truly become them.

Take a sheet of paper and assess yourself on each bullet point, on a scale of 1-10, 1 being I am not like that at all, to 10 being I am super like that and on fire baby! Anything below an 8 and you have work to do, 5-7, you have much work to do. 5 or less, and you need to make big leaps, stop living in fear, get out of your comfort zone and try new, unconventional things. Whatever your score, it's important you pay attention to this list of rockstar qualities and re-

read it on a regular basis to see what criteria you need to not just survive having fibro, but thrive in your life despite it. So please don't put this book down after having read it once and not read it again. Think of this book as your fibro bible; religiously read it weekly, for example every Sunday and use what's in it daily.

PART 2
HOW TO STOP FEELING BAD AND START FEELING GOOD!

CHAPTER 4
BENEFITS AND BLESSINGS OF
FIBROMYALGIA

With fibromyalgia, it's so easy to feel bad, because quite simply your body is full of pain and you have it for life - forever. If you hold on to this negative thought in your mind it is not going to do you any good and you will feel bad, and you want to start feeling good, right?

So how do you start to feel good about having fibro with the scenario I have just filled your head with? Okay, we need to examine the benefits of fibro. *'Did you say benefits? Really? What benefits can there possibly be to having fibro?'* I hear you say. Remember, everything happens for a reason and there is always some positive in every situation, and if you don't think that already, then start believing that because what you put into your mind and focus on expands. Start believing there are positives to having fibro. Fibro has improved my quality of life in some ways and it can improve yours. Do you remember me telling you about the constant flight or flight mode your body goes into when in the presence of an abuser and how this happened to me for 8 and half years with one of my abusers? This applies to if you feel threatened or in danger in any way, and it also applies to if something feels wrong. Fibromyalgia makes you super sensitive to any type of pain. This can be anything from picking up a kettle, that once left a pain impression on my hand even though nothing was visible to the naked eye; to crouching down on my knees on the floor and being in agony for several days after, with pain from those knees – again, no visible marks; to wearing clothes that leave a red mark and pain impression. To any outside person, it would seem bizarre you could get pain from a kettle handle right? But this is fibromyalgia we are talking about, which can seem bizarre and ridiculous to even my own mind at times, so we must forgive the oversight and ignorance on others' behalf, whilst confidently knowing the reality of what actually happens to us, whilst not dwelling on it, but shrugging it off as coming as part of the fibro bundle. You must accept what is, without focusing on it, or paying it any particular attention in these circumstance in which it is playing up. But there are times when fibromyalgia will tell you if something does not feel right and is no good for you, to stop you going into that situation, or to help you to get out of it quicker. This is where the benefits come in and paying more attention to your pain, can help you.

Just like fibromyalgia can make you feel 10 times more physical pain when physically hurt, than a 'normal' person would experience, (so I was told by a doctor), fibromyalgia pain is made significantly worse by negative emotions such as stress, worry, anxiety, depression, fear, upset, hurt and pain, and you are able to notice situations that make you feel this way, a lot more easily than the average person because your body will physically flare up! You could cause these negative emotions, but more than likely they are the result of how you react towards how others treat you. Think of this flare up as a superpower, because with this great insight, you can learn to let go of what does not help you, and in fact hinders you, a lot faster than others. You know you MUST let it go, for your own good, because it is the antidote to cure that flare up of pain on top of your usual pain that you have to learn to live with. You can train yourself to live with your fibro pain, that is within your own control, and so is how you react towards others in terms of your ultimate conscious response, but the way your body will often react involuntarily to danger or threat of any kind and how others behave and act towards you, is not within your control. You owe it to yourself and your wellbeing to stop that pain. This means there will be people who you have to reduce spending time with, give up being in a relationship with, or cut out of your life completely to stop that pain. The relationship between pain and fear is one of great interest to me and so it should be for you. If your pain is greater than your fear of giving up what is causing you that pain, you will give it up. If it isn't, then you won't. You may find other coping mechanisms, but ultimately, you should get out of those situations as soon as possible, for your own health and wellbeing.

Fibromyalgia is a blessing in disguise for me, I see the huge benefits it has brought me and I feel so grateful and thankful for that. It helps me to look after myself better than I did before. I am aware that if I allow a person or situation to induce more pain or worsen my current pain, then that could lead to me being on crutches or in a wheelchair and that is the ultimate threat to my current freedom that I keep reminding myself of. Of course you can adapt to cope with any situation and still survive or thrive within it, but as I currently have the choice to not do things to induce that, I will take that lifeline and save my freedom and know that if I ever do get into that situation, I have no regrets. I won't be, or stay in, a relationship with anyone who is no good for me, however much I may feel for them. I will cut loose people who are bad for me, which is what I would not do in the past. I will now put myself first and lead the type of unconventional teenager lifestyle that I was born to lead and not care what others think, as I only have one life and time is so short and precious. In this way, I feel freer than I have ever felt in my life before. I feel empowered to live for me, to recognise that living for oneself is not an act of selfishness, but rather an act of duty of care to yourself, and an owe-it-to-yourself-to-love-yourself-enough situation. It is fibro that makes me realise how very short life is and how fortunate I am to have such a wonderful life in spite of fibro. I also feel more thankful, blessed, and grateful to be alive. Every day I wake up I feel how wonderful life is, even if something is going wrong or not according to plan and I have tears, I still love life. I am a much more positive thinker, I have to be, or I get more pain as a result. In essence, my fibro punishes me for negativity and keeps me on track for being as positive as possible. Some people are fighting for their lives, while I can still go to theme parks, zoos, aquariums, on days trips, out clubbing – using my 21st Mindset – I will explain more about that later in this book. I actually take more risks because of fibromyalgia and I also take more care about me. I spend more money on living in the now, because of the thought that one day I may not have mobility like I do now, whilst trying to make plans for my future years through creating an online income, so in the future I can work from home full-time and have the money to pay for my care, should I need it. I will not allow toxic people to continue to consume my thoughts – even when they get in there, I will work hard to get them out as soon as possible and know that this time shall pass. I have learnt to react less to others who are hurtful and I have to be around them, such as a person where I used to work, because I know it will hurt me more. When I compare my life now, to before I had fibromyalgia, and I focus on the blessings and benefits of having it, I am able to love my life and myself so much more. It has encouraged me to be at one with my personality, because it hurts me not to be, and I am now my true authentic self so much more, because of it. I really do embrace my quirky, because life is too short not to be who you were truly born to be. I think the less you are like yourself, the more your fibro flares up, as the more you are not being true to who you are and that in turn creates negative emotions that will induce pain. So let me ask you, are you *really* being true to who you are? Are you *really* being your true authentic self? Are you *really* embracing your quirky?

Sometimes with my abusive ex, before I was diagnosed with fibro the year after we split, I would want to go into hospital just to have a break from him. I trained myself after we split, using NLP (Neuro Linguistic Programming), which I had learnt on a Coaching Academy course, to be happy being single, as I did not want the pain of a situation like that, to ever happen to me again. There was a colleague where I used to work, who worked in the canteen and she kept fainting; I saw her passed out on the floor. She was referred to see someone because of 'her' problem. After this repeatedly happened, she temporarily worked on our floor as a sales assistant selling mostly kids and baby clothes and accessories, and she looked like a different person, happy; bubbly; and being her authentic self. Me and another colleague, who had also suffered past abuse, worked out it was a way of her body telling her she did not like the job, that it filled her with dread, and that there was nothing psychologically wrong with her but that her body was shutting down as a way of saying to leave that job as it was no good for her. This is what happens when you are being abused or threatened, or in a situation that is harmful in some way to your energy, existence, or happiness. Your own body is in turmoil and shuts down and you go into survival mode, which is a natural response. Animals camouflage themselves to prevent predators seeing them and eating them. She left that canteen job to work permanently on another floor selling women's clothes and accessories and loved it. She never fainted and always seemed happy. So please learn this lesson, that what you think about and what you feel, and what you are experiencing, directly affects the degree of pain in your body. So to feel good, you need to put yourself in positive situations, so that your body will positively reward you. You need to do a job that you enjoy, or turn something you don't enjoy, into something you do, by seeing the benefits of it to you. If you are feeling worse in your job, it's time to move on. You need to get rid of bad people, and negative situations, and that could include limiting the time you spend with certain people, even family, to make yourself happy and in less pain.

This is the rockstar attitude you need to make you feel good:

- Take responsibility for your life.

- Be a leader, not a follower, and come into your own.

- Stop caring what others think and just do your own thing.

- Give up what does not help you and makes you feel bad, anxious, nervous, sad, or worried, and pursue what makes you happy, confident, energetic, and lively, in spite of what others may think.

- Stop listening to negative people and don't allow yourself to stay in negative situations and be around negative people that are no good for you. If you have to be, learn ways of lessening your interaction with them and lessening your pain.

- Be ambitious, have aims and goals for the future so you have something to look forward to and aim for, as this will take your focus off your pain and give you more fulfilment. Then you must take action to achieve them.

- Be your true authentic self and live your life, your way.

- Be around people who support you in your dreams. Get like-minded 'fans' who really get you and understand what you are about.

Remember this quote:

"Feeling good is the antidote to feeling bad. Feeling pleasure is the antidote to feeling pain. Feeling happy is the antidote to feeling sad. Feeling safe; loved and having faith, is the antidote to feeling fear."

This is my own quote from what I have learnt over the years of studying personal and professional development. Make it your mission to get these antidotes as soon as possible and keep them consistently topped up daily, as medicine for your soul. Remember to generate these for yourself, if they are not already in your life. You are in control of your life, no one is going to hand you these things on a plate, you need to go and get them for yourself. Reduce the negative and gain the positive. Accept that life is a struggle and honour that struggle. It will help you learn, develop, and grow yourself, into the best version of you. If anyone told me when I was younger, that life is meant to be challenging to stretch us and makes us become a stronger person, and that I would be able to deal with any of life's challenges that come my way, because with-in my being and every being, is a super human strength, that is more powerful than you will ever know, and you deserve the best in life, so go get what's best for you, it would have made my life so much easier and happier. If I had been told to trust my instincts, to let go of those who held me back and were no good for me, told it's okay to make mistakes and not be a perfectionist, because that is how we learn to cope and be resilient, it would have helped me incredibly in my life. If I had been encouraged to know that alt-hough different to others, my difference is my beauty and that is a positive thing, this would have given me the strength to leave those that were no good for me, to be confident, self-assured, and have higher self-esteem to not just survive, but to thrive in life, my past would have been so much better, but the past we cannot change, we can only learn from and never dwell on. The present is a gift, because with this knowledge that I have just shared with you, you can now apply it to your current situation and start to move forward with your life. So read back through what I have just shared with you, so you can think about it in relation to your own life. Pay particular attention to the fact that you being different is your beauty. It is your strength and your inner power. It is the superhero coming out in you.

Make the antidotes in this quote, your mission and goal in life to obtain. Remind yourself of what you need to feel by writing down the sentences in this quote or type them up, to use as positive affirmations, and read them aloud to yourself every day when you first wake up, before checking your inbox, or replying to any direct messages, or going on social media: **"Today I feel Good. Today I feel Pleasure. Today I feel Happy. Today I feel Safe. Today I feel Loved. Today, I have Faith".** It's important to emphasise the most important words with capital letters, as it draws your attention to that word more. Some people believe it is harder to read capital letters, but when typing those affirmations up, you can put whole sentences in capital letters if it helps you to retain the information more, because your mind associates capital letters with emphasis of higher importance. I have my morning affirmations typed up in a multitude of colours for each one and they are all in capital letters throughout, and after some time, I can retain what they say as second nature to me. So I can read them out aloud, in order, without looking at them. Also write this quote down on post-it notes and put those notes around your home to use as positive affirmations to help you to think and be more positive in your mind throughout the day. What you focus on expands. Your aim is to feel good as much and as often as you can, to feel pleasure, happy, safe, loved, and to have faith in yourself and your future consistently.

Try this exercise, take six fresh sheets of paper, or get a notebook and a pen, write a title on each one of the pieces of paper, starting with, 'What makes me Feel Good?' The second sheet, 'What makes me Feel Pleasure?' Third, 'What makes me Feel Happy?' Fourth, 'What make me Feel Safe?' Fifth, 'What makes me Feel Loved?' Sixth, What makes me Have Faith?' Time yourself for a minimum of 3-5 minutes for each piece of paper, to write down everything that comes to mind under each of the 6 headings, starting with the first. Don't worry if you give the same answer for more than one of the sheets because this will be positive reinforcement of what is required to get you those things so you can be in less pain. Now go...

Once you have written down everything that comes to mind under each of the 6 headings, you now have a permanent list of how to obtain each one, giving you the direct antidotes to the causes of your pain. Yes, you heard me right; you now have the direct anti-dotes to the causes of your pain. Which means you now know how to prevent it and stop it. So why do you need to continue to read this book? Because there may be things you do unconsciously, that put you in pain, and likely you will not have written all of those down, as 'not dos', such as certain foods you eat and the type of bed you have. We will cover these and far more, such as mastering your mindset, in the pages that follow.

You need to keep these 6 lists and refer to them daily. You should read them after your morning affirmations each and every day, and you can use them in conjunction with your affirmations to make those a reality. You should also plan what you are going to do each day to incorporate as many of your antidotes as possible. Aim to incorporate at least 3 each and every day. If you make a plan and are intentional about getting those antidotes each day, and you follow through with the action to bring them to fruition, you should see an improvement in your quality of life. You should also set a time once a week, for example on a Sunday, so you can reflect on how many of those you achieved that week and what action you are going to take to achieve more of them the following week, or to maintain them. Make a note in your diary, and/or on your calendar, that every Sunday from now on, you will reflect on your antidotes and how well you have put each of them into practice over the last week and what action you will take to do more of them the following week. Go do that now! If you don't mark it as a thing to get done, and give it a date on which to do it, you won't do it.

KEY POINTS TO REMEMBER:

Your difference is your beauty.

Don't let your limits limit you.

Practise these antidotes daily using your 6 lists:

"Feeling good is the antidote to feeling bad.

Feeling pleasure is the antidote to feeling pain.

Feeling happy is the antidote to feeling sad.

Feeling safe; loved and having faith, is the antidote to feeling fear."

Say these powerful affirmations to yourself, everyday you wake up: "Today I feel Good. Today I feel Pleasure. Today I feel Happy. Today I feel Safe. Today I feel Love. Today I have Faith."

To combat fibromyalgia pain, have rockstar qualities and attitude. Live with purpose, see the benefits of having fibromyalgia and face your fears using your antidotes.

One of the blessings of fibromyalgia is it makes you super sensitive to all types of pain, including stress and anxiety, and the benefit of this is that you are able to see and feel far quicker, situations that are no good for you and increase your pain, as your body will literally flare up, so you know you need to get away from that source of pain as soon as possible and can do this quicker than other people who can't see this so easily for themselves. You owe it to yourself to do that, and not blame other people and things for not getting away from it, as you have now become consciously aware of it. You become more consciously aware of situations that cause you pain, by taking a mental note of what you are doing at the time; what you are consuming; who you are talking to; and what you are thinking about that is inducing your pain, then you have to have the guts to take that choice and decision to go do something about it now, sooner, rather than later. Which may mean leaving a relationship that is no good for you, cutting contact with certain people in your life that are no good for you and limiting your time with others.

CHAPTER 5
HOW TO OVERCOME
DEPRESSION

If you get, keep, and use, all of your antidotes on a consistent basis and develop a rockstar attitude, you should see your anxiety levels reduce, and therefore your pain decrease as a result. The same goes for depression. If you currently have depression, you should see a lift in that depression, as depression cannot live in the same space as feeling good; feeling pleasure; feeling happy; feeling safe; feeling loved, and having faith. It is the absence of these things and the presence of low self-confidence, low self-esteem and low self-worth, which lead to depression. Along with loneliness, which is often due to a lack of self-love; misunderstanding; being misunderstood; and a lack of connection to others, which is often due to an inability to relate to others, either because you are not around like-minded people, or because you lack the necessary social skills and/or communication skills; or because you lack empathy or emotional intelligence and you can work on those areas to improve them, so there is a solution. You may be an anxious person and worry about what others think of you, but if you were around like-minded people who accepted you for who you are, you would feel more comfortable and safe and be able to relate to others more. If you don't currently have anyone you feel safe around, then find local groups in your area, online and offline, such as through meetup.com; that you have things in common with, and build a relationship with them, and at least one person within them. Remember, if you are meeting just one other person, to always meet anyone offline, in a well lit, public place, and video chat with them first for safety. In order to improve your social skills, guess what? You need to practise being in more social situations. No one in the world gets good at social skills unless they put themselves in social situations. Start off by being social with just one person, who understands you and who you feel safe with. As your confidence grows, build up to being in social situations with 2 people, then 3, or more. It takes baby steps to change your life but you can do it. If you practise your antidotes and are in a happier place in your mind as a result, you will be a more cheerful person to be around socially. Overcoming depression starts with working on your inner core being first. Because if we rely on others for our own happiness and external factors instead of our self, we make our self vulnerable and in an unsafe and insecure position, because our happiness is dependent on the whims and emotions of others, and other factors that could change, such as a job or house, and not of our self. We can only be in control of our self.

Feeling loved is not just about others loving you, but first and foremost about loving yourself, because you are the only person who has to live with yourself 24/7, 365 days a year, forever. The only person you ever truly need to love is yourself, because you live with you and you die with you, so if you don't love yourself, you are a bit stuck! If you don't love yourself for whatever reason, even if others do, you're still not going to feel loved like you would if you loved yourself and you won't be happy. Instead, you will be torturing your mind with your negative thoughts about yourself and feeling you are worthless and not good enough. Just imagine spending every day of your life with someone who you dislike, who you hate, and who you don't want to be around; if this sounds like you, I understand you, as I was that person. Whilst I did not fully hate myself, I liked my hair for example, and at 15 I liked my talkative nature even when others didn't; I disliked myself and felt bad about myself a lot of the time, but most of all I hated my life many times, I did not see a point to it and I wanted to die, I wanted my life to end and the agony of living to stop. If you are feeling suicidal then please don't harm yourself in any way, know you are loved, and seek professional help with a doctor, counsellor, therapist, or other qualified professional, to work through any issues you are facing both past and present. If you live in the UK, Ireland, Scotland, or Wales, you can call the Samaritans to get some emotional support 24/7, visit Samaritans.org for more details. If you live elsewhere in the world, you can contact Befrienders Worldwide, who offer a helpline at limited times in certain countries, visit befrienders.org for more details, and don't forget to use Google to find out about local organisations that may be able to help you in your local area. I had counselling for years of my life in the past. I had both Cognitive Analytical Therapy (CAT) and Cognitive Behaviour Therapy (CBT), and there is no shame in it. It was only when a counsellor asked me to go home and do something I had never done before, to list all of my strengths and all of my weaknesses that I could think of, that I was able to come up with a long list of both. Although I think the negative was a stronger argument than the positive, I was able to see that I had some positives about me and became more consciously aware of that, which sparked a little bit of curiosity about myself and self-love in me. But my self-love journey began one day when I asked myself a logical question about me, "Are you going to not like yourself forever and go around making yourself feel bad to be with you for the rest of your life, or are you going to do something about it, because your life is only going to be a miserable one if you don't?" This is when the penny dropped that I had control of that, at a time when I did not feel in control over a lot of the other aspects of my life, and that was empowering! I realised I was in control and responsible for my own happiness in regard to the way I viewed myself and I would only have myself to blame if I did not acknowledge that and adjust my life accordingly in some way. So I made myself work out what weaknesses I could accept about myself as they are, either because they are not that bad and I can live with them, or that in some ways they can actually be positives. And I began to ask myself if those things that I did not like about myself or I saw as a weakness, really were, or if it was other people telling me they were, and they were forcing their opinion on me about myself, as if it were a fact! Yes, I found at least a few of the latter! Any weaknesses and negatives that made me hate myself, or my life in some way, I knew I had to change and would have to find out how to do that but live with them as they are for now, whilst being a little loving towards myself that at least I recognised them and wanted to do something about them. These days I am forever trying to improve my life and myself. Sometimes I manage to do it and make a ton of progress and change myself and my life, others times I still struggle to get all the answers and make that change, but I still love myself for being willing to learn, explore, develop, and grow myself as much as possible, and really there is no point in giving myself a hard time about it when I still feel I can't make that change, because the only one that will suffer in the long run, is me, so I just have to love all of me, as I am. And I would love you to do the same and do what I did.

It's time for a self-assessment. Take 4 sheets of paper. On one write the heading, 'What I Like About Myself'. On the second sheet write the heading, 'What I Dislike About Myself'. On the third sheet write the heading, 'My Weaknesses' and on the fourth sheet, write 'My Strengths'. Now time yourself for a minimum of 3-5 minutes for each piece of paper, and write down all the corresponding answers. Do not worry if you repeat any answers on another sheet of paper. Be honest with yourself and make sure you write something on every sheet.

One you have finished writing your answers, take the things you dislike about yourself sheet, and your weaknesses sheet, and see if there are any similarities in your answers. Oftentimes, we can find that what we dislike about ourselves, we also believe are our weaknesses, although this is not necessarily the case, it could be our own perception of it, as what one person dislikes, another could love. Now I want you to go one step further, and on a scale of 1-10, I want you to give each answer a number. 1 being it is not impacting my life and 10 being it's causing huge problems in my life. So for example, if you have social anxiety, on a scale of 1-10, how is that affecting your life? If you don't need to be sociable for your job and you can go out when needed then that may be a score of 3, but if it is causing you to miss out on seeing friends and enjoying life and you feel depressed because of it, you may give yourself a 10. I want you to do the same for the what you like about yourself sheet, and your strengths sheet. I want you to compare if there are any similarities in your answers, then give yourself a score as before, on a scale of 1-10, but this time I want you to grade yourself on how much you like your likes about yourself, 1 being I like it a little and 10 being I love it, and how much you play to your strengths, 1 being I hardly use that strength, to 10 being I use that strength a lot. So if for example, on the sheet of paper you wrote about what you like about yourself, you included, "I am intelligent", how much do you like that about yourself on a scale of 1-10? And if you wrote that same thing down as a strength, how often do you use that intelligence on a scale of 1-10?

Once you have every answer graded, for those you gave yourself a 7-10 score on the weaknesses and dislikes about yourself, I want you to write down what specific things you are going to do to change and improve that. What are the steps you will take and act upon? If you don't know how, Google it! Google has the answer to almost anything at your fingertips. Or borrow a book from the library; ask a friend who has already achieved that, how they did it. And write these methods down as to how you are going to improve that. So for example if you lack confidence, type into the Google search bar, 'how to be more confident' and select what answers resonate with you the most and take action on them. You also need to reflect on what weaknesses and dislikes you can accept about yourself rather than change. In other words, your action would be self-acceptance, and how you will achieve that self-acceptance. You need to be bold and brave and make that decision, right here and now, that you either accept it as a weakness or dislike, at least for the time being, or you are going to change it and decide how. You can't say to yourself I hate this and live in a perpetual state of dislike or hatred for yourself, or towards yourself, because of it. If you do that, it's only going to put your emotional and mental health in turmoil as you are going to be constantly at odds with yourself and that will cause more pain in your body. You need to be decisive and make a commitment to yourself, to show yourself the love, self-acceptance, and self-respect you need and deserve, right here and now.

Of the things you like about yourself, and are strengths, anything below a 5, meaning you like it less than average about yourself, or you use that strength less rather than more on average, I want you to write down how you are going to increase liking that about yourself and how you are going to use that strength more on a daily or weekly basis, so that you are using it more times often than not. So if for example intelligence was a strength and you liked that about yourself, you could increase your intelligence level further and make it a greater strength and like it more, by taking an online course in a subject you want to know more about and you could do some of that course daily, or every other day. Or you could do an in person course at college or university. Whatever age you are, it's never too late or too early to change the direction of your life and do something for yourself to improve yourself and your life in some way, in fact it is essential for your own health and wellbeing and to decrease your personal pain which in turn decreases your fibro pain. Do you see now, that by making changes to your life and by focusing on improving your self, your fibro pain reduces as a result? This is the truth about fibro. This is what you need to do to improve your energy, feel happier, and have less pain.

So if you have done this exercise correctly, you should have a plan of actions for working on your strongest weaknesses and dislikes about yourself, so you can change them, or accept them. Also a plan of actions to increase your strengths so they become stronger in your life, and a plan of actions of how to like yourself more. Now is the hard part. Now is the time you have to go and put those into action. And I don't mean tomorrow, or a week from now; I mean right now. Your brain has a way of talking you out of things that seem threatening, and getting out of your comfort zone is uncomfortable and threatening to your current life, but it's something that is essential to your growth and will improve your confidence and self-esteem going forward, which can only be a good thing.

A lack of ambition, goals, dreams, and hope for the future can also cause depression. That's why it's so important you get into a habit of developing yourself and self-improvement, so you have purpose and meaning in your life. Your job is to be the best version of yourself, and to constantly seek to improve yourself and your life. If you get all these antidotes and develop a rockstar attitude, where you are going for your goals, ambitions and dreams; you will do what you love in spite of what people think; you will be your true authentic self, you will love yourself and have others love you because you will be around like-minded people who love you for who you are, who understand you, and love being connected to you, this will deplete your depression and make you feel good. If you do not have any goals, ambitions or dreams, you are wandering around in this big world with no direction or meaning, and no life purpose, and that should now become your meaning of life, to search for that purpose, everyone has one, you just have to be open to finding it and have to go on a journey of self-exploration to get it. Just think of what fun you will have discovering it. If you go back to your six lists of antidotes, amongst your lists you should see where improvements need to be made, either because you have written down the answers to the 6 questions as to what you need to do and you realise you are not currently doing them, or because they are missing from your life and you have not noted them down as things you need to be happy, feel pleasure, feel good, feel safe, feel loved, and to have faith. If you have not got much on your lists to help you to feel and experience these antidotes, make this your priority to work on over the coming months and challenge yourself to add something new to each list once a week for at least the next 6 weeks! Sit down, every Sunday (or a day of your choice), and force yourself to reflect and write down something for each of the 6 lists for the next 6 weeks. As there are 6 antidotes, you will need to think of 1 way of obtaining each, so in one week you will have come up with 6 solutions. Write down in your diary, which day for the next 6 weeks, you are going to do this, and put it on your calendar, go do that now before your mind talks you out of it, then stick to it and do the work; you will be so happy you did!

KEY POINTS TO REMEMBER:

Depression is caused by the absence of these antidotes in your life:

"Feeling good is the antidote to feeling bad.

Feeling pleasure is the antidote to feeling pain.

Feeling happy is the antidote to feeling sad.

Feeling safe; loved and having faith, is the antidote to feeling fear."

Along with loneliness; misunderstanding; being misunderstood; and a lack of connection to others, which is often due to an inability to relate to others, either because you are not around like-minded people, or because you lack the necessary social skills and/or communication skills; or because you lack empathy or emotional intelligence and you can work on those areas to improve them. Also, a lack of self-love and no direction or life purpose can cause depression.

To overcome depression, you must work on any of the areas of your life just mentioned that are problems for you, and get, keep, and use, all of your antidotes on a consistent daily basis, and plan each and every morning how you are going to incorporate at least 3 of those antidotes into your day, for that day. If you sort your problem areas out, you should get your antidotes, and if you work on your antidotes, it will help you to sort out your problem areas. So for example if you feel sad and lonely because you don't have any friends, it could be you have a problem relating to others and one of the antidotes you have on your list is to be around people who understand you, as it will make you feel good, loved, and happy. So note down what actions you are going to take to find these people, such as join online forums or closed groups on Facebook to join in the conversation and make friends. Join groups who you have something in common with, or find local offline meet-up groups in your area through a reputable organisa-tion such as meetup.com, and then make the decision to take action and make contact with them. Go join some online groups, do it now! And if you meet up with anyone in person in the future, always meet strangers in a public place! If you are meeting them alone, rather than in a meet-up group, insist on Skyping them first – or if they won't video chat with you in some other way, such as through Google Hangouts or Face-book, forget it! If they have issues with that, it's their problem, don't risk it and make some other friends. Human beings still need human, in person, offline contact sometimes, so endeav-our to always have both online and offline friends in your life.

If you are feeling suicidal seek professional help with a doc-tor, counsellor, therapist, or other qualified professional! If you live in the UK, Ireland, Scotland, or Wales, you can call the Samaritans to get some emotional support 24/7, visit <u>Samari-tans.org</u> for more details. If you live elsewhere in the world, you can contact Befrienders Worldwide, who offer a helpline at limited times in certain countries, visit <u>befrienders.org</u> for more details, and don't forget to use Google to find out about local organisations that may be able to help you in your local area.

Read the next two chapters to find out more ways you can over-come depression!

CHAPTER 6
WHAT TO DO IN AN ABUSIVE SITUATION

If you are in an abusive situation, or around abusive people, this will make you feel depressed, anxious and stressed, and greatly increase your fibro pain. I am not a trained counsellor, or therapist, and not professionally qualified in the area of abuse. All I can do is tell you what to do based on my own experience and knowledge, so always, always, seek advice from a professionally qualified person as I cannot guarantee the outcome of what I am about to share with you, as I am not in your circumstance and I don't know what your abuser is capable of.

There is a wealth of knowledge and resources on the internet about what to do if your life is in immediate danger, such as remain as calm as possible, including in your tone of voice, and do whatever you can to stay safe and alive, this may mean complying with your abusers wishes and giving them what they want, and try to get away, get to safety, and call the police as soon as you can. But every circumstance is different and may require a different response, especially if you are being threatened with a physical object, and that is beyond the scope of this book so please look for qualified and reputable advice about that.

ABUSE AND DYSFUNCTIONAL FAMILIES!

So what if you are depressed because you are in an abusive situation, that is not immediately life threatening, or you are part of a dysfunctional family that make you feel worthless or useless about your life and yourself?

In this case, do not blame yourself, but be aware of the situation and get outside help and know that it's even more of a reason why you must try to love yourself, so you can be as mentally strong as possible around these people. Although it's not your fault, only you can take responsibility for yourself to either get out of that situation which I would always recommend, or be able to cope with it in the most safe and least damaging way as possible both mentally and physically, if you feel compelled to stay for whatever reason; such as because you are financially trapped. Know you are not responsible for others' behaviour, only your own. If you are constantly feeling belittled and worthless, told you are crazy, stupid, and that no one will love you for who you are, and are mocked for being you by those nearest and dearest to you, especially on a consistent basis, I know what that is like, to not feel loved, valued and appreciated for who you are. I know what it's like to be mocked, to be put down a lot of your life and made to feel small and that other things are more important than you and that any decision you make is the wrong one. All I can say is you have to remain strong and know that these people have their own problems that they are projecting onto you, seek as much outside help and support as possible; talk to friends if you can, or talk in private online support groups and forums to not feel so alone. Get a counsellor; therapist; or get other qualified help, and try to get out of that situation that is causing you pain and misery as soon as possible. Never believe that no one will love you for who you are and that you are worthless, because it simply is not true. You are not worthless; you are worthy of love and a good life. You are fully capable of love and of having others love you. Those who say you are crazy and stupid, are the ones who are behaving so. Abusers, narcissists and controllers, want to manipulate you, to make you feel bad about yourself, so they can throw you off balance to make you feel unsure of yourself, so you always need them as your emotional crutch, and they can push you away again at any time.

So if you are living at home with someone who is not good for you, then I understand how hard it is not to be depressed, but you owe it to yourself and your fibro, to release yourself from that stress and agony in your life as soon as possible, that is no doubt making your pain so much worse. It creates bad energy in your body that can stay with you for years to come as trauma, which causes fibromyalgia and maintains and sustains the agony and flare ups of fibromyalgia. You need to set yourself free from all past and current trauma as much as possible, the more you do this, and get and apply your antidotes, along with eating the correct foods, eliminating the trigger foods that traumatise your body because they are no good for it, and do everything else I explain in this book, the more you will feel calm, happier, in control, have far less swelling and flare ups and the more you are able to love your life in spite of your fibro. In the meantime, be a superhero to yourself, by giving yourself a mission of constant self-protection, self-adoration, positive self-talk, and of feeling valued to be alive. Take note of how well you are coping in that situation and praise yourself for dealing with it over and over again.

FOLLOW THIS SUPERHERO PLAN

Spend the least amount of time possible with those toxic people, by trying to make outside in person friends and healthy online friends, but be careful not to get drawn to other controlling people without realising it. People who have had, or are in, abusive relationships, tend to have a habit of getting into others, as they find it hard to know what a good relationship or friendship looks like and they seek validation and a feeling of self-worth that is not within themselves, or has never been instilled into them. And if you are not getting the love, care and attention that you naturally want at home, it means you will be seeking it elsewhere. This is why getting those from yourself is super important for self-protection, otherwise you can be easy prey for predators. Don't feel so scared by this that you never try to make friends with others, just know that some people are trustworthy, and some are not, and online they can cover up their lies more easily, but take your time to feel and sense if someone you grow attached to quickly, really does have your best interests at heart, or if they are using you or have alternative unhealthy intentions. Use your intuition to judge people in this way and be guided by it.

Get a counsellor or therapist you like and get on with, who makes you feel good about yourself and you feel can help you – but realise only you can take the action to remove yourself from the situation you are in!

Find and join online private support forums and groups of people who understand what you are going through, but also find groups of people who have recovered from abuse and are leading a good quality of life, as this will help you to know that you can have a better life.

Find and join private online groups of people who are an inspiration in some way, as well as those who are doing the hobbies you like, or who like and enjoy the same things as you do and have shared interests. This will help you to feel less alone, more optimistic for your future, and valid as an individual.

Keep a diary of your thoughts and feelings, this will help you to not bottle them up which is toxic for your body and soul!

Make your diary your best friend and make any pets you have your best friend too. That way, you can have some friends if you don't have any, and if you do have friends, it will help you to feel less alone when they are not around.

Start a blog. A blog is great therapy for the soul. It can distract your mind, get you interacting with people on other blogs and you can share your photos, daily ideas, and thoughts, but remember a blog is not private so only post stuff that you know will not lead you to any harm, and don't post anything that may be subject to libel. A blog will also let you feel in control of something, when the rest of your life may feel out of control, and this is empowering.

Get outside interests and hobbies as much as possible. Fill your mind and life with as many inspirational books, people, and videos as possible, and work on obtaining and applying your antidotes, despite those toxic people around you. Think of your antidotes as your super shield and force field against the darkness and evils of this world. If you are still a child in the eyes of the law, ask yourself if it's possible you could go and live with another family member who you love and trust, and who does not make you feel bad about yourself.

Don't forget these types of toxic people want to make you feel weak and powerless so they can control you and put you in a situation where you feel you can't leave, because if you did, you would be worse off, but it the long run, you would be better off, even if it will be hard at first. It took me 18 months to 2 years to get over my abusive ex, but it was worth it, because I have both my financial independence and my freedom for the rest of my life, from that mental prison he put me in! I did a 3-month pattern-changing course, with a company called S.A.F.E. that stands for, Stop Abuse For Everyone, to recognise patterns of behaviour in people who are likely to be abusers, to avoid being with a guy like that ever again. It was one of the best things I have ever done in my life and if you get the opportunity to do that yourself, I highly recommend it. My doctor in the UK referred me to it. I am sure what I learnt in that course has saved my life numerous times over, so I can recognise and cut a bad guy or person out of my life quickly. As I also said before, I have my fibro as my weapon against getting with anyone like that ever again, because any signs of an abusive guy, then I get him out of my life in a shot, even if I really like him and it pulls on my emotional heart strings. My fibro will not let me be with or stay with, someone who is bad for me, as my intuition kicks in, my anxiety shoots up, and my pain levels become unbearable. It's my superpower in the fight against those potentially abusive relationships!

In a nutshell, to stop depression, you either have to change the way you think about yourself and your life and accept yourself for who you are and your situation for what it is; or change yourself; or change your life and situation in some way and keep making changes until you are happy with it and just choose to be happy and positive regardless, because the alternative is more painful if you don't. You have nothing to lose by choosing to be happy and positive, but you have a lot to lose if you don't. You have to take active responsibility for yourself and for your own health and wellbeing, by making a decision to change yourself, your mindset, and your life! I used to dislike myself and my life and have a very passive attitude towards it and not value my worth, now I am the opposite, I love my life, I love myself implicitly; even with my weaknesses and flaws, my life is always quirky and there is never a dull moment when I am spending time with just me!

HOW TO EMBRACE YOUR QUIRKY AND NOURISH YOUR SOUL

In 2012, I developed my "Embrace Your Quirky" philosophy to overcome depression, and I apply this to every aspect of my life. I want to share it with you to help you break free from depression in conjunction with what I have previously said to you. Embrace Your Quirky means to always be your true, authentic self, regardless of what anyone else says; thinks; or does. If you are in a dangerously abusive environment, you may not always be able to be the true you because survival is a must, but keep reminding yourself of this philosophy and if you live on your own or are in a healthy relationship and home environment; live as you, and for you, and be free, because you soul will thank you for it. If you are doing things that are in tune with your values, morals, and beliefs, you will lead a healthier, happier and more fulfilling life for you. If you do things that you know go against your own beliefs, that don't feel right, that you know you are faking because of peer or societal pressure, or that you feel obliged to do to keep someone else happy, you won't feel good and that will cause you pain in your inner being and manifest itself in your body! Which is what you don't want to happen and must prevent. I know people who are depressed and anxious because they are so worried about what people think of them, and they will say things to please others or keep quiet about their true feelings so as to avoid hurting others, or being rejected. I learnt a few lessons in life about this; the one who has the loudest voice in a given situation tends to win, regardless if what they are saying is right or wrong and the harshest lesson being that these people will not care about what happens to you when you are gone from this world, so why worry about them and what they think while you are alive? Life is too short! Ask yourself; do you want to experience the full joys of life while you are here to live it, or would you rather pamper to everyone who comes along in your life, and live a life out of reaction? This is how you can get put upon, how you can get used and abused, and believe me, not everyone in this world is going to like you anyway, there will never be a time when you can please everyone, and why would you want to? That is like self-abuse for the soul, because you are not valuing your own self worth. You are in effect saying what others think, want, desire and believe, is more important than what you want, think, desire and believe, that their life holds more value than your own and it puts them on a pedestal. This is not going to make you feel good, happy, safe, loved, and secure within yourself, and you need to be! You want to have the least amount of pain possible in your life, and that means in every sense of the word and every aspect of your own being. You need to nourish your soul with things that make you feel good, alive, energetic, and that you're thriving! Not let others run your life, persuade you, and dictate to you! Go live your life for you and be free! Embrace Your Quirky and love every little weird, strange, and incredible thing about you! Self-love is the number one most powerful tool in your own ammunition against the evils of this world and those who are trying to dominate, control and own you! Own your life, and own yourself! Take responsibility for yourself and be your own mother and father to you! Look after yourself, as if you were your own child! Adore you, because you are worth it!

KEY POINTS TO REMEMBER:

If you are depressed because you are in an abusive situation, if your life is in immediate danger, remain as calm as possible, do whatever you can to stay safe and alive, this may mean complying with your abusers wishes and giving them what they want, and try to get away, get to safety, and call the police

as soon as you can. But as every circumstance is different and may require a different response, especially if you are being threatened with a physical object, look for qualified and reputable advice about that, as I am not qualified in such matters.

Never believe that no one will love you for who you are and that you are worthless, because it simply is not true. You are not worthless; you are worthy of love and a good life. You are fully capable of love and of having others love you.

Abusers, narcissists and controllers, want to manipulate you, to make you feel bad about yourself, so they can throw you off balance to make you feel unsure of yourself, so you always need them as your emotional crutch, and they can push you away again at any time.

Living with someone who is abusive, makes your pain so much worse. It creates bad energy in your body that can stay with you for years to come as trauma, which causes fibromyalgia and maintains and sustains the agony and flare ups of fibromyalgia. You need to set yourself free of all past and current trauma as much as possible to help reduce your fibro pain and flare ups.

If you are living at home with someone who is abusive towards you in other ways, such as using manipulation or control, then follow this plan:

- Spend the least amount of time possible with them.

- Give yourself a mission of constant self-protection, self-adoration, positive self-talk, and of feeling valued to be alive.

- Obtain and apply your antidotes as much as possible, despite these toxic people, because they are your defence against those who are trying to dominate, manipulate, and control you.

- Get a counsellor or therapist you like and get on with.

- Realise only you can take the action to remove yourself from the situation you are in and try to do that as soon as possible!

- Ask yourself if there is anyone else, such as a family member you could go and live with.

- Get outside interests and hobbies.

- Find and join online private support forums and groups of people who understand what you are going through, but also find groups of people who have recovered from abuse, as well as those who are doing the hobbies you like and who have the same interests.

- Write your thoughts and feelings in a diary and make that your best friend.

- Start a blog, but remember it's public.

- Use the pain of your fibro as your superpower and force field against the evils or this world, to ensure you stay out of abusive relationships in the future.

To stop feeling depressed in general, use my Embrace Your Quirky philosophy to be your true authentic self, no matter what anyone else says, thinks, or does. Stop worrying about what others think of what you do, and value yourself more, remember, these people won't care about you when you are gone, so why worry about them while you are alive? Life is too short and precious for that and so are you!

CHAPTER 7
HOW TO HAVE MORE ENERGY AND ZAP
DEPRESSION WHERE IT HURTS!

I am different to most people with fibromyalgia in the sense I have a ton of energy. I am naturally a hyper, bubbly and energetic person, and have not let fibro get the better of me in that respect, although I could have done. Since having fibro I feel I have more energy in my life, and if it starts to deplete, I know how to fix it. Such as through music, movement, and doing things that make me feel happy and alive every day. Having a happy list helps with that. If you haven't done that yet, go do that now and write down at least 10 things that make you happy. On my list, I have included taking a hot shower, going to the cinema, listening to dance music, and eating allergy free ice-cream. I need to top-up daily with doing things that make me happy, to prevent depression ever returning. I practise daily being grateful and thankful for the small things in life and I trained my mind to be happy being single using NLP (Neuro Linguistic Programming). Yes, you can retrain your brain to be happy, providing you take action and get into new habits and patterns of thinking. I can live on my own happily, as my true authentic self, but when I was in a bad relationship, I couldn't do that. When you are not being true to who you really are in your heart and soul, when you are not aligned with your mission and purpose – when you don't even know your purpose, you will wander around in life with little hope, with a sense of where do I belong in this world, depleted energy and lethargy, and this will cause depression. There was a time in my life when I was miserable, I felt and looked older because I was living my life as a result of circumstance and societal expectations and conventions, in an environment that was no good for me, and I did not know my life purpose; I was depressed – never again. That way of life does not suit me. A 'normal' life is not for me, but an extraordinary life, is where I want to always be. Now I am living life my way, I have far more energy and I am so much happier. Yet, like anyone else, if I focus on any pain, or any negative emotion, this is when my energy starts to wane. So let me ask you again, are you living your true and authentic life? Are you really being true to who you are? Or are you living as a result of circumstance and societal norms and expectations? And please allow your inner intuition to answer; allow your heart to feel those words and allow your mind to decide the truth from that feeling and emotion.

To quote the World's Leading High Performance Coach; New York Times Best Selling Author, and one of the most watched and followed Personal Development trainers <u>Brendon Burchard</u>, "The power plant doesn't have energy; it transforms one form to another. It generates energy and transmits it. We are the same. You don't "have" happiness; you generate it. I say if you are going to generate any form of energy let it be joy and love. Let that be your intention and the lights come on."

What you put into your mind, directly affects your thoughts, feelings, emotions, and actions, which impacts the state of your body and your levels of energy. So from now on you need to be mindful of what you consume, what you watch, listen to and read. You need to be prepared to give up that which does not energise you or make you feel good, pleasure, happy, safe, loved, and have faith. Let's take the news for example, particularly on TV; it's full of murder, rape, violence and destruction. Let me ask you a question, does watching the news make you feel good, pleasure, happy, safe, loved, or have faith for the future? So why are you watching it? Why are you consuming it and allowing it to consume you? Because you will feel you are missing out if you don't watch it? Hmmm let's see, you will be missing out on negativity from rape, violence, murder and destruction ... yeah, why on earth would you want to miss out on that? I mean, that is definitely going to make you feel good, happy, and give you pleasure, right? Think about it... Oh, you grew up being taught that is what you NEED to do; it is essential; you would not want to miss the news, how on earth are you going to know what is going on in the world! Do you really need to know? Food and water is what you need to live, you don't need to watch the news. I don't watch the news and I am not just alive but thriving because of it. Why would you NEED to know about violence, murder, rape and destruction when you already know they happen? So by watching these things each day, you are compounding these things happening over and over again in your mind, and instilling a deeper sense of pain within your soul, which in turn causes you more emotional pain and therefore body pain. If you were conditioned from a young age that you must watch the news, this can be fixed. Being conditioned from a young age is about habits that have been instilled into you, often by your parents, so you need to get out of the habit of watching, reading, and listening to the news, and put a new habit in place for at least 21 days for it to be long enough that you will stick at it. This requires you to be disciplined and force yourself to be uncomfortable for a while, with not doing something you have done for a long time. Yes, you have to force yourself to not pick up that paper, or switch on the radio, or the TV, and make yourself do something else. Be aware, that you are in charge of your life, no one else. Not your parents, not your spouse, and not your offspring. If they want to watch that and they live with you, go into another room, watch an inspirational video on YouTube, go outside and smell the flowers, do something that makes you feel good, happy, and gives you pleasure, you don't have to do what they do, you are your own person. Think about what else you watch that is negative and apply those same disciplines. Soaps for example, are purposefully dramatic and play on your emotions to get you hooked. The producers have to keep thinking of the most heart-pounding storylines to grip you! Have you ever found yourself getting angry, upset, feeling pain for the characters so much that it seems like you know them and they are a daily part of your life? Maybe you shout at the TV, or you cannot believe he cheated on her yet again and you discuss this with your friends over breakfast, and you just have to find out how long it will go on for THIS time, before she realises!! You cannot miss an episode, because you want to be there for the big reveal! In essence you are an addict, these soaps are your drug, and you are at the mercy of these negative emotions that will have an impact on your mind, emotions, and body pain! I admit, I was a soap addict and I was an addict of other TV shows. As a general rule, I gave up watching TV a long time ago and feel so much better for it. I occasionally watch movies on Blu-ray and I enjoy watching films at the cinema and the whole magical feeling that the cinema creates for me, it gives me a lot of pleasure and a buzz of excitement, which makes me feel revived, refreshed, and re-energised. But I am also very consciously aware of how the content of those films emotionally impact me and if it is a negative or positive experience.

The relationship you have with yourself is super important for creating energy in your life and managing your pain. So let me ask you a question, are you currently living your life for you? Or are you living your life for others, or how you THINK they would be happy for you to live it? Take 5 minutes to write your answer down in relation to your daily activities, the people you associate with, and your goals, ambitions and dreams. Now is the time to look at those answers and reflect upon them and ask yourself, are you *really* where you want to be in life despite your fibro pain? Your pain is always going to be present in some way, but the trick is to live your life for you in the most positive; vibrant; energetic; authentic way possible, to reduce your pain and lead a better quality of life and not let your fibro stop you from doing anything you want to in life. So are you doing that? Are you doing what you want to do, regardless of your pain, are you pushing through it, or are you saying, "I am in too much pain to do that?" If you want to live your best quality of life, you will need courage. Courage is not just about acknowledging your fears; it is about facing your fears head on and pushing through them; feeling the fear and doing it anyway. If you keep saying, "I am in too much pain, I can't do it", then guess what? You just deepened that negative emotion, wiring it into your brain even more, making you feel helpless and hopeless and that will zap your energy. So are you living your life for you, or at the mercy of your fibro pain? Are you being a fibro victim, or a fibro warrior, leading the way in your own life? When you look at your ambitions, goals and dreams for your future, are those truly your own? Do they make you feel energised, alive, and vibrant? Or are they really what your partner, spouse, or family member would want you to do? Are you afraid to do something crazy like set up your own business because it's something you have never done before and your friends or partner tell you, "That's the craziest thing I ever heard, why would YOU want to do that? I think it sounds too risky and you have no experience of that anyway!" If you have nothing to look forward to that enthuses you, give you pleasure, freedom, and happiness, you will have no hope for the future, and that will zap your energy and make you feel small. In order to have more energy you need to do things that will get you out your comfort zone and stretch you, expand your mind, and give you new possibilities. You need to have things in your life to give you hope and allow yourself the gift of faith that everything will be okay, despite your fibro; that you can still live a deep, meaningful and extraordinary quality of life! Are you allowing your life to be at the mercy of others' behaviour and what they think? Are you living a life of action or reaction to those around you? If you are always at the mercy of others' agendas in your life, your life is not your own and your precious energy is being consumed in ways that is draining you, not lifting you. You need to find and do things that lift you, not drain you. Learn to say no to others and protect your precious energy.

Be purposeful on what you focus on, otherwise you can fatigue your brain, and if you are putting negativity into your brain, what do you think will happen? It will zap your energy and cause you mental and emotional upset, and therefore physical pain. Take proactive steps to focus on what will make you have a positive mental and emotional state, and stop reacting to other people's negativity. Let me ask you a question, do you find yourself on Facebook, consuming news feeds of other people's problems? Of their dramas? Of their hate for those who have done wrong to them? If you do, it's time to let go of that and refuse to get mixed up in it for your own good, go on their profile, and click that "following" button, to switch it off so you should stop seeing their posts in your news feed. You don't have to de-friend them, but if they have no meaning or purpose in your life whatsoever, then you don't need them to be your friend, so unfriend them. Not everyone is always going to be positive in life 24/7 and that includes me. We all need people who are there for us when things take a turn for the worse and if we are not there for them when that happens, we cannot expect the same in return. It is always important to spend some time in your life giving to others; in fact, it can be great medicine for your own soul, to help that of others, it can be rewarding and give you that feel good factor dopamine hit. So I am not saying to avoid speaking to anyone who is negative, the trick is to speak to those who do not want be in that situation; who want to improve their life and will take steps towards doing so, and they are just going through some tough stuff. And even then, sometimes, you have to put yourself first if you are becoming in a worse state because of it, or you are going through some things in your own life that means you are not in a strong state to help others at that point in your life. Fibromyalgia makes you super sensitive to pain and this includes emotional too, so if you have a high degree of emotional intelligence and you have a deep empathy with others and can feel their pain, their problems can have a negative impact on you emotionally, which can decrease your energy and increase your body pain. What you must avoid doing, is paying attention to those who are just always being negative for the sake of it, who get a buzz out of it, who love the attention and the drama. If you must check in with certain people who are negative, do so knowing that their drama is not yours, that you are there as a friend to listen, and help if you can, but if you feel your energy levels depleting, make your exit and do what you need to do to get your energy levels back up again.

Be sure to surround yourself with as many like-minded and positive people as possible. You can choose your friends, but your can't choose your family. Be sure to choose friends who make you feel positive and great, who are supportive and understanding, who encourage you to be the best version of yourself that you can be and whom make you feel good, just by being around them. If someone makes you laugh, smile, and feel good about yourself, then spend more time with them to help with your energy boost. If someone is making you feel bad about yourself, or bad when you are around them and giving off negative energy towards you, they are no good for you, so cut them loose. If your family is negative, tell them how their actions and behaviour is affecting you, if they won't listen and respect you enough to take you seriously, limit the time you spend with them.

Ensure your environmental surroundings make you feel energised and alive. Make sure that the rooms of your home are full of things that are beautiful to look at and wonderful to touch, so you feel good being in them. Whether that means a favourite painting on the wall, a cuddly teddy bear on your bed, flowers on your dressing table or wallpaper that makes your feel all warm and fuzzy, it is essential you get this right for you. It's no good if you are staring at a brown carpet wishing you had blue. It's no good living in a minimalistic environment, if you feel better having lots of stuff around you. And it's no good having lots of stuff around you if you feel claustrophobic, and you need to de-clutter your environment to make way for new energy to come into your life. If you have got lots of things from the past that hold bad emotions for you and therefore bad energy, letting them go can make way for much more positive energy to come into your life. You could sell those items and use that money to redecorate your home in a way that makes you have positive energy. And ensure the temperature of your rooms makes you feel good. I work better in heat, but sometimes I feel more tired, lethargic, and lack energy when the heating is on, so I have to open windows to keep myself alert to stop me from falling asleep. So if you have the heating on in the winter and you are feeling more tired; drained, and lacking energy, have you considered it may be the heat causing that? A lack of oxygen can also cause you to feel lacking in energy and so when there is less oxygen in the room, if you have the windows closed for example, you could feel more tired and sleepy and it could be that, not your fibro that is actually making you feel that way. This equally applies to if your breathing is shallow and lacking in oxygen, which is a symptom of anxiety. I sleep with the window open even in winter now, as I sleep better with that extra amount oxygen I am getting.

If you have sleep problems and close the windows at night, try leaving them open and have hot water bottles in bed and extra blankets on top of your duvet to stop you getting a cold.

You may also feel tired, lethargic, and lacking in energy, if you eat foods that are hard to digest, as digestion requires a lot of energy to break down the foods you consume. On the other hand, you may not be eating enough of the foods that give you energy such as fruit, particularly bananas, which are a good source of potassium, but be careful of bananas as I discovered they can naturally lower blood pressure, which is no good if you suffer with low blood pressure, but a great thing to eat if you suffer with high blood pressure and want to try reducing it. I can't say it will work for definite but it's always worth trying and see how you feel as a result, as everybody's body is different. You may not be eating enough protein, such as almonds or oily fish that also give you those vital omega 3s to reduce your fibro body pain, and certain vegetables, particularly green leafy veg like spinach, which is also a good source of potassium! We will be talking more about foods to eat and not eat in chapter 13 and it's essential you explore what foods give you energy and what foods deplete it, so you have the right energy levels to maintain and sustain you throughout the day. Did you know if you are allergic to sugar; sugar can zap your energy? Certain hot drinks can make you feel sleepy and less energetic, such as a milky drink or some herbal teas.

If you are overweight, don't get much exercise, or you have bad posture, all of these can make you feel tired, exhausted, and lacking in energy. Being dehydrated can also make you feel tired and lacking in energy. Unless you are taking certain vitamins that turn your urine yellow, your urine should be clear if you are getting enough fluids. If it is dark yellow, you are dehydrated and need to drink more water; filtered or bottled mineral water is best, and 2 litres a day minimum is best to stay hydrated and alert and awake. I was recommended to drink 2 litres of water a day when I went to the hospital for a bladder problem. So pay attention to these things and take action to stop or rectify these whenever needed.

Although it appears unknown if those who have fibromyalgia have anxiety and depression because of it, or as a symptom of it, it stands to reason that if your fibro is caused by trauma, which I mentioned at the beginning of this book as being the cause of mine, and I believe many others' too, it is likely you would have become depressed or anxious about what caused your trauma, even if you are not consciously aware of it. So you need to repair that unconscious damage because it will store and manifest itself as bad energy and create pain in your body. Know you cannot change the past, but you need to work on subconsciously releasing it and letting it go, for your own good, to get a better future. Go for counselling if it will help you, and start getting into personal and professional development to change your life. If you keep doing the same thing, you will always get the same result. Will this require work and effort on your part? Absolutely. But this is crucial to your growth. If you grow and develop yourself, it will give you more meaning and life purpose and that will make you feel better mentally and emotionally, which in turn will increase your energy and decrease your conscious pain. Both subconscious and conscious bad energy, need to be replaced with good energy, so you can have more energy in general. If your body, mind and soul, is full of bad energy, that leaves little room for good and positive energy.

Connection to others is essential to not feeling depressed, which will zap your energy. If you are an extrovert, you will feel alive and energised by being around people who are like-minded and positive, so make sure you set dates and times in your diary for meeting up with these people so you always have something to look forward to, to get you out and about. Join groups to make more friends but also just by going into the town or city and being around others, rather than spending too much time indoors by yourself can give you an energy boost. If you are somewhat intro-verted, although you may prefer your own company in general, and you can feel drained of energy if you are around people too much, you can get depressed if all you have is mostly yourself for company. It is only natural as a human being to need some connec-tion to others for mental health and wellbeing. So get out and about; socialise and make some new friends. Google groups in your area, go on www.meetup.com to find groups to join and meet up with. Try to join groups that will be a mixture of your interests and that will grow you in some way. If you are feeling down, don't stagnate in your own introverted company; go meet up with those positive friends or like-minded people; go do what lifts you up; or go try something different to grow yourself.

Change your state, and you change how you feel and think. Re-member that rockstar attitude? Go listen to your favourite positive uplifting music, and move your body to change your state. It will give you more energy; make you feel alive and happier. Keep a list of your top 10 favourite positive songs that make you feel ener-gised whenever you listen to them, so you can play them whenever you need an energy boost or energy top-up!

Focus your mind on your goals, ambitions and dreams, and start taking action to get them. If you don't know what those are, make it your mission to find out, to discover your purpose, and to find your 'why' in life. Set some goals as to how you are going to dis-cover your purpose – which usually lies in what you are passion-ate about, what enthuses you, and what hobbies and interests you have. When you make progress in your life and start achieving things however big or small, you will gain momentum and motivation. Your self-confidence will increase; you will have a higher self-esteem, more self-worth and self-respect, more satisfaction and fulfilment, and more joy in your life. That in turn makes you feel more alive, energised, and improves your quality of life. Thereby decreasing your stress and anxiety levels, making you feel great and in less pain. Go live for you. If you are living your life as others would want you to, you will never be happy and at one with your soul and this will cause you more pain and zap your energy and make you feel like your life is not your own, which is the opposite to what you want and need.

Having the right frame of mind when you wake up will instantly make you feel more alive and energised for the day ahead. This should start with an attitude of gratitude. By stating out loud things you are grateful for when you wake up, you will set yourself up for a positive day ahead. Positive self-talk is key to improving your daily happiness and vitality, and giving you good energy. Follow a morning practice of gratitude, along with saying those morning affirmations that I mentioned in a previous chapter, **"Today I feel Good. Today I feel Pleasure. Today I feel Happy. Today I feel Safe. Today I feel Loved. Today, I have Faith"**. Remember to consistently reflect and evaluate how you are feeling. Notice what you are saying to yourself on a daily basis; are your words to yourself empowering, encouraging and supportive and making you feel alive? Or are they negative, disempowering, and expressing disbelief in yourself and your own abilities, making you feel small and helpless? If you are not feeling good about yourself as a whole, you need to change that because no one else is going to do it for you. Don't wait for someone to come into your life and give you permission to change it and be happy, because change has to happen from your heart and being to make it stick.

Best-selling Author and Motivational Speaker Mel Robbins, sums up the fundamentals of creating more energy in your life. "Being energised is not to do with what's hard or easy, it has to do with what expands you or shrinks you. Make decisions with your heart and soul. Ask yourself does the decision you are about to make, expand you? Expand your future? Expand the possibilities of your life?"

Use the Quick Fire Checklist you are about to read, on a daily basis, to make sure you are on track and stay on track to getting and sustaining more energy within yourself and your life.

Quick Fire Checklist Of Dos and Don'ts For Creating More Energy Within Yourself and Your Life!

- Don't focus on your pain or think about it. As pain is a negative emotion it will drain your energy.
- Do whatever it takes to distract your mind and focus on positive things.

- Don't stay around negative and depressed people.
- Do be around positive people who inspire you and lift you up.

- Don't get caught up in other people's problems! That will drain your energy.
- Do focus on creating solutions to your own problems!

- Don't blame everyone else for your problems or the way your life is!

- Do take full and sole responsibility for your own life and the way it is!

- Don't focus on what other people have in life and feel envious or like you are missing out.
- Do focus on your own life, on how to obtain the things that you want and what makes you happy.

- Don't live in fear!
- Do push through your fears and develop a fearless attitude!

- Don't dwell on the past and about negatives things that happened and wish you could have changed them, as this will zap your energy!
- Do have a positive mental attitude towards life. When you reflect on the past, accept it as it is and that you did the best you could at the time. Let go of any guilt you may be feeling or holding onto, and see the positive outcomes from it and what lessons you learnt, which in the least is that you are a stronger person because of it.

- Don't have a negative, pessimistic, or cynical attitude towards life now or towards your future.
- Do foster a positive attitude and mindset for the present moment, as well as for your future!

- Don't do work that is mediocre and that won't keep you engaged and active.
- Do work that you can be deeply engrossed and engaged with!

- Don't think what is the point to life.

- Do find your life purpose. Think about what you like, love, what makes you feel energised; inspired; motivated; invigorated, and alive, and what you are passionate about, and go do that as much and as often as you can, every single day of your life.

- Don't live without any future plans, goals, ambitions and dreams, as this will zap your energy because you will have little hope and faith for the future.

- Do think deeply about your own life and envisage a compelling future, and revisit this future every morning and day. Be optimistic that the future holds good things for you and that you can get through anything life throws at you! Set goals, ambitions and dreams for your future, with a plan of action of how you are going to achieve each one of those and take action to achieve them, because if you don't they will only be just a paper exercise! Believe you are born for a special purpose and act like it.

- Don't bottle up negative emotions otherwise they will consume your thoughts, feelings and actions, and this will zap your energy.

- Do foster positive emotions and make them a habit. Get your thoughts, feelings and emotions out in a constructive manner, such as by writing them down in a journal or diary, or by blogging!

- Don't consume negative content – books, articles, TV, music, news!

- Do consume positive content, such as personal development books and courses, educational videos, motivational and inspirational content.

- Don't stay stagnant in life and watch endless amounts of TV and spend endless amounts of hours playing video games and waste hours of your precious life on un-meaningful activities that won't grow or develop you to be the best version of yourself. Whilst these may make you feel good and are enjoyable to you and give you some degree of pleasure, there are other more meaningful things to do, which will give your life more purpose and meaning, making you have more energy and zest for life!

- Do limit the amount of time you spend watching TV and playing videos games, do them less frequently, cut the amount of time you do them, and devote some of that time to personal and professional development and ensure you are continuously learning, developing and improving yourself. Do meaningful activities that will improve yourself and make you the best version of you. Then do something that will help others, change people's lives in some way, or improve it, as this will make your life feel more worthwhile and give you an energy boost.

- Don't stay in bed all day!
- Do get up and get dressed, even if you don't feel like it.

- Don't live a life of satisfying others' agendas. Learn to say no to requests that will not help you in your own life; goals; ambitions; dreams or mission.
- Do deeply engage with your own life. Live a life taking action, and of go-getting your own hopes, ambitions and dreams, and stick to the path of your own mission.

- Don't wake up without intention and lack meaning for your day. Don't give your energy away at the start of your day by going on social media and answering emails and messages as soon as you wake up, or make others' priorities your own. There are only so many things you can do in a day, or in a set period of time, and everything you do takes energy. If others take more of that time than you do focusing on yourself; on your own wants and needs, it means you will have little energy left for yourself to achieve those.

- Do get up and before you do anything else have a large glass of water, say your positive affirmations, review your lists of antidotes and plan your day and how you want it to be. Include as many of your antidotes as you can and include things that will help you to grow and develop yourself in some way! Wake up with purpose, intention, and direction for your day ahead, to create your ideal day every single day! Set your own priorities for that day and a minimum of 3 goals to achieve by the end of the day, and ensure you achieve them by taking action!

- Don't look back in life with regrets about everything you did not do because you were at the mercy of others each day and what their needs and wants are, leading a life of reaction to those around you. If you are feeling that your life is at the mercy of others, you won't feel energetic, vibrant, and look forward with positivity to the rest of the day.

- Do live your life for yourself and not for others. Work on your own personal and professional development, educate yourself, take courses, go to seminars, read educational books, and actively participate in changing your life and yourself! If you feel your life is full of things you most look forward to and want to do, it will motivate you for getting your morning off to a great start and for the rest of the day. Motivation and taking action on your plan for the day, builds momentum; that in turn creates energy!

- Don't focus, or dwell on the negative in any situation, or say, "Why has this happened to me?"
- Do focus on the positive of every situation and believe everything happens for a reason and think what the reason may be in a positive way! Ask yourself, "What did I learn from this?" Or "What benefit or advantage is there to this happening?"

- Don't not exercise at all.
- Do exercise such as walking, gentle stretching or aerobics. If you are in a wheelchair, wheel yourself to the shops or around a park or do chair aerobics.

- Don't do exercise you know will cause you to be in much higher pain for many consecutive days.
- Do keep pushing yourself beyond your comfort zone that little bit more to see if you can get a bit more exercise into your life. Even if you know it will cause you some pain, still do some exercise! Non-movement causes lethargy!

- Don't stay in one spot and not move around. Don't listen to slow tunes and quiet music! This type of music may help you to chill out or calm down, and send you off to peaceful sleep, but it won't give you an energy burst or make you feel energised!
- Do bounce on the spot for a quick energy burst and do get up and move around as much and as frequently as possible, more than you would usually do. Even if you are indoors a

lot, move about, dance around your home to positive, up-beat, energetic tunes, such as dance music, techno music, power ballads, high-octane pop music or powerful rock tunes. Even if you are in a wheelchair, move your hands above your head to positive, upbeat, energetic music. Wheel yourself around your home and try to do as much upper body movement as possible, because motion creates energy! If you want to be in PJs all day, just make sure you are up and moving around as much as possible and don't be in PJs all day every day!

- Don't stay indoors all the time.
- Do get out and about and get some fresh air into your lungs.

- Don't isolate yourself from others.
- Do join online and offline groups and meet up with people in person, not just online, and at least take a walk in a place where there are people.

- Don't live in an environment that is negative or no good for you.
- Do live in an environment that makes you feel vibrant, alive, happy and energised!

- Don't live off junk food or eat stuff that you know is not good for you. Don't starve yourself and don't eat a stodgy meal or fatty foods.
- Do eat foods that energise you. Eat a lot of raw foods such as broccoli, spinach, and fresh fruit. Eat regular healthy meals. Eat healthy snacks! Nuts are meant to be energising if you are not allergic! Eat more protein and less carbs for more sustained slow release energy and to help prevent

you from becoming overweight. However, if you have low blood sugar you may want to eat small amounts of carbs throughout the day to keep your energy levels up!

- Don't use being overweight as an excuse for your decrease in your energy, even though it may be one of the causes!
- Do either lose weight and/or love your size you are. There are still plenty of overweight people who have a ton of energy, including those who dance, because they do things to create their energy!

- Don't breathe shallow, as this will cause a lack of energy and fatigue.
- Do breathe deep as this will get more oxygen into your body, which will increase your energy levels. Practise deep breathing exercises daily.

- Don't get dehydrated and have yellow urine.
- Do stay hydrated throughout the day, drink at least 2 litres of water a day and make sure your urine is clear.

- Don't do anything that is not in line with what you love, what your heart and soul desires, what feels good to you, or your intuition tells you will be no good for you!
- Do create experiences that will energise you; nourish your soul; enrich your life; connect you to others; make you feel enthusiastic and alive! Listen to your intuition and do what your heart desires, what you love, and what will be good for you! Where emotion goes, energy flows, so do things you feel an emotional pull towards or attach an emotion to it!

- Don't have negative self-talk and believe things are impossible, as this will drain your energy.
- Do believe you can achieve anything you put your mind to, have positive self-talk on a daily basis, and keep telling yourself, "You can do this; you got this; keep going!"

KEY POINTS TO REMEMBER:

You don't have energy and happiness; you generate it!

Don't be around negative and depressed people who will not make you feel any better or positive about life, even if you are depressed yourself – depression and negativity breeds depression and negativity! Be around positive people who inspire you and lift you up; who are energetic and enthusiastic about life, as energy and enthusiasm is infectious!

Practise daily gratitude. Be thankful and grateful for what you have each and every day of your life! Remember there will always be someone who is worse off than you.

"Ask yourself does the decision you are about to make, expand you? Expand your future? Expand the possibilities of your life?"

Create a happy list of at least 10 things and fit as many into each and every day of your life as possible.

Create a list of at least 10 of your most energetic, vibrant, positive and uplifting songs, and fit as many into each and every day of your life as possible to energise you.

Don't get caught up in other people's problems, focus on creating solutions to your own problems!

Take ultimate responsibility for your own life and don't blame others for any problems you may have.

Wake up with purpose, intention, and direction for your day ahead, to create your ideal day, every single day!

Don't get caught up in other people's agendas and start answering messages, emails and texts, first thing in the morning! Start your day right with gratitude, and these morning affirmations, "Today I feel Good. Today I feel Pleasure. Today I feel Happy. Today I feel Safe. Today I feel Loved. Today, I have Faith. Plan and prioritise your day ahead to include 3 goals that will help you achieve your ambitions and dreams! Then act on them!

Don't think about your pain. Distract your mind by doing things that make you feel enthusiastic, alive, inspired, motivated, energised, and that are in line with your own beliefs, intuition, and what your heart desires!

Eat foods that energise you and drink at least 2 litres of water a day.

Breathe deeply. Exercise, move, walk, dance around your home, bounce, and get out and about.

Stop consuming negative content, on TV (including the news), in books, magazines and in music! Listen to positive upbeat music to energise you. Watch motivational and inspirational videos, get into personal and professional development and do things that will develop and grow you in some way each day. Educate yourself, take courses, go to seminars, read educational books, and actively participate in changing your life and yourself!

Foster positive emotions, stay positive, believe everything happens for a reason and don't dwell on the past but forgive yourself and look forward to your future with a positive mindset and attitude!

Don't allow your life to be at the mercy of others. Live for you, put your energy and focus on what you want in your life, and act on that!

Do work that you can be deeply engrossed and engaged with!

Motivation and taking action on your plan for the day, builds momentum; that in turn creates energy!

Where emotions flow energy goes! So live your life with purpose, be intentional, and do things you feel emotionally attached to!

Believe in yourself and that you can do anything you put your mind to!

Have positive self-talk on a daily basis, and keep telling yourself, "You can do this; you got this; keep going!"

CHAPTER 8
HOW TO INCREASE YOUR
CONFIDENCE

Confidence needs to come from within your own being, not from external factors and the validation of others. If your confidence comes from those things, then you will always be left in a vulnerable and fragile state, as those things can be changed without warning and you have no control over them and will feel powerless as a result. The more confident you are in your own life, the less anxiety, worry and stress you will have, and the less pain your body will be in, which is the ultimate goal.

Do things in spite of your pain and you will see an increase in the amount of things you can do, which in turn will raise your confidence and self-esteem. You have fibro, so accept you will have pain from it but remove that pain from your conscious thought and focus on what you want, like and love, and go do it, otherwise you will miss out on life and life is for living!

Realise you have the power of choice in every aspect of your life and that you are in ultimate control of your life, no one else, and especially not your fibro. Fibro may be a part of you, but it does not own you, always remember that!

Choose to be confident and act like it. Even if you don't feel confident, acting like it will help you to become it, because you are practising for it to become a reality.

Develop more positive body language. Hold your head high and walk strongly and boldly.

Speak with certainty and clarity, don't mumble or hesitate in your speech.

Stop worrying about ifs, whats, mights, and maybes.

Believe that you are worthy and capable.

Believe in yourself and in your ability to work things out, even if you don't know how at the time. Know you can cope with anything life throws at you.

Be intentional about who you are. Be crystal clear about your own identity. With intention, comes confidence and momentum, which builds energy. Be who you are and show that to the world.

Embrace your quirky, by allowing yourself to think differently and act differently and by being your true authentic self, regardless of what anyone else says, thinks, or does.

Stop caring about what others think of you and the life you lead.

Speak your truth and not what others would want you to say.

Accept that not everyone will like you and stop trying to please everyone.

Realise that life is too short to not do what you want in your life and that your life is your own.

Honour the struggles of life and see any obstacles as challenges that you will gladly accept and overcome – say to yourself, "bring it on!"

Accept it is okay to make mistakes, but believe there are no failures in life, just lessons you learn from and therefore there is nothing to fear, which means you can take more action.

Force yourself to get out of your comfort zone. Be decisive and courageous, and make the conscious decision to try new things despite any fears or worries you may have. Stop thinking about your pain, and instead think about you enjoying yourself and the benefits to your confidence and self-esteem of trying something new and challenging in your life. Reassure yourself that you make good decisions and look for evidence to support that; of when you have made good decisions before, and also of when you have done something that caused you pain, but you coped and overcame it, so you can be confident you will recover again, should the worst happen.

Don't dwell on doubts and fears and keep repeating them in your head. Instead, think and visualise what the more positive outcome could be and pay attention and focus on that.

Take action to do things you are passionate about.

Do more of what you love and less of what you don't.

Learn to see change as a good thing.

Increase your strengths.

Learn to laugh at yourself and don't take yourself too seriously otherwise you can get upset, especially in those fibro fog moments. My fibro brain decided it wanted to change the names of people I had worked with for years, to something it believes was the right name for them, it's weird, but hey I am quirky, so I can do weird, and if I didn't laugh about it, I would cry, so I always choose laughter every time.

Develop more competencies in areas of interest to you. Increase your knowledge and develop skills and abilities in those. The more you grow competent in those areas, by practising those skills and abilities that you have learnt over and over again, the more your confidence will increase!

Be around people who support you and believe in you, your skills and abilities. Cut or limit your time with those who don't. Get rid of naysayers and if you can't, don't pay any attention to them.

Have friends who are positive and open-minded, who respect you, who value your worth, and who want you to do well in every aspect of your life. If you feel you are putting far more time and energy into the friendship, you care far more about them than they do about you, or you feel less like yourself in it and more like you are just going with what they want or going through the motions, it's time to speak up about it and get some new friends. Although you can get many friends in principle, always look to get a few quality true friends that will stand the test of time with you, those that see you at your best, and also support you at your worst.

Don't rely on other people to fulfil your wants and needs, take ownership of those for yourself!

Learn and practise self-dating. Go to the cinema on your own; out for meals on your own; day trips; weekends away; and do as many activities as possible by yourself. Be intentional about this. Schedule time in your diary for these dates and write them on your calendar and ensure you keep your dates with yourself no matter what. This will give you a huge confidence boost, because it will increase your self-love, self-worth, and self esteem. It will bring you closer to your own soul and increase your independence and self-reliance.

Tell yourself positive affirmations every morning as soon as you wake up and believe them.

Pay attention to the words you are saying to yourself. Change any negative thoughts into positive ones and give yourself positive self-talk throughout each day. Praise yourself for your efforts, for your achievements – however big or small, and realise just how awesome and amazing you are. Give yourself a hug and lots of love.

KEY POINTS TO REMEMBER:

Realise you have the power of choice; choose to be confident and act like it.

Be decisive and courageous, force yourself to get out of your comfort zone and try new things in spite of any fears or worries you may have. Don't focus on your pain, instead focus on enjoying the challenge of trying new things. Look for evidence of when you have tried something new, and that caused you pain, but you overcame it, so you can reassure yourself that you can recover, should the worst happen.

Self-date and do as many things as possible by yourself!

Develop more competencies in areas of interest to you. Increase your knowledge and develop skills and abilities in those.

Have intention of who you are; be your authentic self and show that to the world. Speak with certainty and clarity. Speak your truth and not what others would want you to say and do not care what others think.

Believe in yourself, your abilities and capabilities, and act like it.

Be around people who support you and believe in you, in your skills and abilities, and cut or limit your time with those who don't.

Use positive self-talk on a daily basis! Tell yourself positive affirmations every morning as soon as you wake up and believe them.

Honour the struggles of life; see obstacles as challenges you will overcome.

Believe there are no failures in life, just lessons you learn from and therefore there is nothing to fear, which means you can take more action.

CHAPTER 9
HOW TO DECREASE YOUR ANXIETY
AND WORRY LESS

Anxiety is excessive worry. It is common for people with fibromyalgia to have depression and anxiety. Whether their anxiety is a symptom of their fibro or they have anxiety and depression because of it, is not clear. I was diagnosed with GAD Level 4, (Generalised Anxiety Disorder), some time before my fibro diagnosis and have experienced anxiety in my life since childhood. But you read at the start of this book, it was after my fibro diagnosis that I became free of depression, which I had also experienced most of my life. My fibromyalgia was the catalyst for change in my life. They say it takes a big event in your life to force you to change and this was one of those huge moments, because it forced me to change my mindset to a positive one and start to work on me. The thought of me being in a wheelchair or on crutches for the rest of my life was a much greater threat than the pain of continuing to let my thoughts be consumed in a negative way. I knew I had it for life and I either saw the positive in this situation or what would be the consequence? Pain and debilitation! No thank you!

If we talk about being in pain, and think about it, we will experience more of it, as we are bringing it to our conscious thoughts. So that is why sometimes when we worry and we worry that we are worrying, that in turn creates motion, it gives energy to what we are worrying about and makes it have a bigger impact on our life, whereas if we had just thought, 'that's a worry' and let it go, that worry would have no hold over us and we can keep moving forward in our life. Worrying is something we do to avoid getting hurt, but it also creates a situation of pain that may not be there in the first place. So choose your moments of worry wisely and let go of those worries that are just there for the sake of their own existence.

To quote my Grandma, "You die if you worry, you die if you don't, so why worry?" She had a point. Worrying does not fix the problem, but it can make it worse in your mind.

Some techniques I have found to help me worry less, which can help you are:

> Don't think about your pain and the fact your fibro could get worse, but instead focus on living life to the max, on doing as much as possible, and living as vibrantly and energetically as you can! Live for now with no regrets but still focus on a good future for yourself doing what you love and think positive!

> Make yourself feel safe. I had nightmares for years of my life and I did not realise it was due to me not feeling safe. With all of the abuse I've had; the distrust from unhealthy and bad relationships, it's understandable, but it wasn't until I became consciously aware of this that I could do something about it. I knew nightmares are often based on anxieties and fear, but I could not pinpoint it to these two words of 'feeling safe'. As soon as I recognised this, I was able to put something as simple as "I feel safe", into a morning affirmation that I read out loud every day along with my other affirmations as soon as I wake up, and also as part of my 3 affirmations I attach above my door handle, to the inside of my flat front door, that say, "I'm Safe, I'm Happy, Life

is Good". This is so not only do I feel safe in the morning and for the rest of the day while in my home, I also feel safer out of it. I can truly say this has made a huge difference to my life, so now I am no longer as fearful of going to sleep and feel so much safer. When I am out, I remind myself, "You can look after yourself, you are strong; you can deal with anything that comes your way, you are okay, I believe in you!" I try to avoid any potential unsafe situations but I also try not to live in fear. It helps I have quite big muscles for a girl, that I like to keep toned through my few morning press-ups for keeping my back strong and pulling my large shopping trolley full of food.

Practicing gratitude. Every morning wake up feeling happy and thankful to be alive. Think how lucky you are to be alive when some people have taken their last breath. Before going to sleep, write down 5 things you are grateful for, proud of, or that make you happy. By being thankful and grateful, you are switching your mind from a worried focus on negative issues, to focusing on the positive.

Celebrate successes however big or a small. This could be anything from taking the rubbish out, getting up and getting dressed, to winning an award, or flying around the world. At the end of each day, write down 5 of these successes, and create a success jar that you fill up with pieces of paper with your successes written on them, so at the end of the year you can empty that jar and celebrate just how successful you have been. Use as many jars as you like.

Distract your mind with fun and positive things.

Listen to music that makes you feel naturally high, due to the tune, words, or feeling it creates within you. Music about overcoming things; getting back up again after falling down; about working harder and smarter; and about reaching for the sky or stars; are all fantastic.

Going out on self-dates, to the cinema and for a meal, is great for your soul and can really get you back in touch with your inner being; with who you are; your life purpose; and what you want to become. This positive focus will take your mind of your worries and make you feel good!

Laughter is one of the greatest forms of natural medicine as it's hard to feel sad or depressed when laughing, and worries and cares leave your mind. Meet up with friends who you know make you laugh whenever you see them, or watch a movie at home that makes you laugh out loud.

Meeting up with friends or family, and chatting to them on the phone can really help if they are positive about your future and reassuring you that everything will be okay.

Write down problems and feelings in a 'worry diary', so you can offload them and stop bottling them up. It will make your mind clearer, and feel less cluttered and better.

Brainstorm solutions for how you could overcome your worries and then choose which ones to action.

Change your mindset to see every obstacle as a challenge that you will gladly strive to overcome.

Take ownership of your decisions and be more decisive.

Honour the struggle of life. Realise you need that struggle in order to stretch, develop, and grow yourself, otherwise you will just stagnate in life and become depressed and bored with it; you will feel like you have no meaning to life and that will become your struggle.

Believe everything happens for a reason and trust your intuition and allow yourself to be led by it.

Focus on your future. Pursue your passions, ambitions, and dreams, so you feel hopeful, have faith, and are reminded of the skills, knowledge, experience and special qualities you have, so you feel better.

Keep saying to yourself, "I will be okay", and resolve not to panic, as it will only cause you more pain and not solve the problem.

Give up watching TV and the news. The media is designed to create drama and provoke an emotional response, often an upset or negative one, which brings doubt and unresolved problems to your mind so you feel compelled to carry on watching to get answers and closure. If you don't watch it, you retain your emotional power and energy – which is so badly needed to keep your pain levels to a minimum. If you don't give into it, you won't be affected by it.

Worrying is designed to protect you, but often it just makes you sicker. Whenever you worry, if it is not a life-threatening situation, acknowledge that worry and say to yourself, "thanks for sharing," then let it go.

Delay worry by saying, "I will worry about that later", and either you will forget about the worry completely, or you can bring it up again, only at a dedicated worry time. So if you worry daily, plan to set time aside each day, at a set time, to allow yourself to worry and offload.

Stay positive, because worry instils fear and negativity into you, and feeds off of them. By instilling positivity into you, through affirmations and positive self-talk on a consistent basis, you can counteract these negative emotions and worry less, thereby decreasing your pain.

Praise yourself regularly and say, "You are doing great".

Get out of your head and enjoy the moment.

Adopt a stop-thinking-and-start-doing attitude. Make this your motto, "Don't think about it, just do it!"

You will notice that some of the things that help me to worry less are the same or similar to, those that stop me from being depressed and help me to create more energy in my life and sustain it. This is because the things that make you feel worried, nervous and anxious, are often the things that contribute to your depression and zap you of your energy. Stop those things and you nip depression in the bud and raise your energy levels!

KEY POINTS TO REMEMBER:

Don't focus on your pain and that your fibro could get worse, instead focus on living life to the max, on doing as much as possible, and living a vibrant and energetic life right now! Fo-

cus on a good future for yourself doing what you love and think positive!

Choose your moments of worry wisely and let go of those worries that are just there for the sake of their own existence.

Worrying does not fix the problem, but it can make it worse.

Think 'that's a worry' and let it go.

"You die if you worry, you die if you don't, so why worry?"

Make yourself feel safe. Put "I feel safe" into a morning affirmation and read it out loud every day, along with your other affirmations, as soon as you wake up. Attach an affirmation above your door handle to your front door, that says, "I'm Safe, I'm Happy, Life is Good".

Practise gratitude. Every morning you wake up feel happy and thankful to be alive. Before going to sleep, write down 5 things you are grateful for, proud of, or that make you happy.

Celebrate your successes however big or a small.

Distract your mind with fun and positive things.

Listen to music that makes you feel naturally high.

Write down problems and feelings in a 'worry diary'.

Brainstorm solutions for how you could overcome your worries and then choose which ones to action.

Change your mindset, to see every obstacle as a challenge that you will gladly strive to overcome.

Honour the struggle! Believe everything happens for a reason and trust your intuition and allow yourself to be led by it.

Focus on your future. Pursue your passions, ambitions, and dreams.

Keep saying to yourself, "I will be okay", and resolve not to panic.

Give up watching TV and the news.

Delay worry by saying, "I will worry about that later". Or bring it up again, only at a dedicated worry time.

Stay positive, praise yourself, and use positive self-talk on a consistent basis.

Get out of your head and enjoy the moment. Make this your motto, "Don't think about it, just do it!"

CHAPTER 10
OVERCOMING FEARS AND APPLYING
YOUR ANTIDOTES

I am going to throw you into a bit of a wobbly now. Because there are times when you will have to overcome your fears by tackling them head on. I know if I get stressed, anxious, or nervous, that my fibromyalgia pain will get worse. A lot of these feelings are brought on by fears; fears of the unknown; fears of what ifs, and fears of being in certain situations. I also know that to overcome fears, I have to force myself to do things that are uncomfortable for me at times and anxiety inducing, but the reward of getting through that challenge, will make my life less painful in the long run. The more we do something that is uncomfortable, the more we get comfortable with it, which increases our competence and confidence. Remember, the antidote to feeling fear; is to feel safe, loved, and to have faith. So whenever you are faced with a fearful situation, you have to put thoughts of feeling safe and loved in your mind and you have to have faith that you will get through whatever challenge you are faced with. Remember, you are a rock-star warrior; you can do anything you put your mind to. You live with pain. You are amazing, incredible, and very gifted, and you can survive and thrive in any situation.

In April 2017, I went abroad for the first time ever on my own, by Eurostar, to Disneyland Paris. I was in a state of anxiety over this, but I knew that arriving at that destination and the amazing time I would have there, outweighed my fear of either missing out as none of my friends could go with me, or 'potentially' being in danger, because of recent terrorist attacks taking place in Paris. I was due to arrive the day the president of France was to be elected. This meant as well as the risk being highest due to that, security would also be on super highest ever alert and so there was a degree of safety in that thought. Remember, what we focus on expands and what words we put into our mind creates meaning and feeling, which shapes our reality. My goal was to feel the least anxious as possible and to reduce the potential fibro pain I would experience as a result. So I had the choice to focus on the 'potential' danger, which was a threat to me, or to focus on the high security, which made me feel somewhat safe and comforted. It was important that I used the word 'potential' danger, as that made it less 'fixed, definite' danger, and more of a 'might be' dangerous, which was a weak argument in comparison to the super high security that would be on 'super highest ever alert'. So I went, even with some anxiety that I had been able to reduce, with so much joy and happiness in my heart and mind, that the most beautiful place I had ever been to in my life, I would get to experience the magic and pleasure of once again. Remember, the antidote to feeling sad, is feeling happy; feeling pleasure, is the antidote to feeling pain; and feeling joy and happiness makes me feel good, which is the antidote to feeling bad. I also phoned my mum when I arrived at the Eurostar terminal, before I got my passport checked prior to boarding Eurostar. This meant I felt loved, which is part of the antidote to feeling fear. I already felt the safest I could with the highest ever security. And I just had to take that leap of faith, that no matter what life throws at me, I can and will deal with it. Faith is the final part of the antidote to feeling fear which can also be the scariest, as it relies on yourself more than anything, but you should radiate love for yourself and believe in your own abilities, no matter what. So I had all the ingredients of my antidotes in place. So this is how you can apply that quote and your antidotes in real life situations, to reduce or prevent your fibromyalgia pain flaring up. The last time I went to Disneyland Paris before that, was with my cousin in 2014, she was used to going abroad by herself and with others. Whereas I hardly ever go abroad, because I don't like flying on a plane and have no desire to go travelling. Yes I have a fear of flying, more like petrified of the part where I am in the air – I feel like I am falling backwards, and if my desire to travel outweighed the fear, it may be different, but right now, just to go abroad by myself is a huge leap forward of progress for me, so I am pleased with myself about that. It's important to note, you must recognise and acknowledge your achievements however big or small, to give you the courage to face more fears, to reduce or prevent more long-term pain, and live a more fulfilling and abundant life. Remember, life is short, don't wallow in the bad stuff. Like a superhero, use your armour of antidotes as your super weapon against the pain you need to decrease and not bring to conscious thought.

Which leads me nicely onto the next chapter, the power of conscious thought.

KEY POINTS TO REMEMBER

Short-term pain for long-term gain: There are times when you will have to overcome your fears by tackling them head on, and force yourself to push through them by doing things you are uncomfortable with, that challenge you, but that will make your life less painful in the long run.

The more we do something that is uncomfortable, the more we get comfortable with it, which increases our competence and confidence.

Remember, you are a rockstar warrior; you can do anything you put your mind to. You live with pain. You are amazing, in-credible, and very gifted, and you can survive and thrive in any situation.

Like a superhero, use your armour of antidotes as your super weapon against the pain you need to decrease and not bring to conscious thought.

PART 3
MASTERING YOUR MIND!

CHAPTER 11
THE POWER OF CONSCIOUS THOUGHT

The most crucial thing to managing your fibromyalgia and decreasing your conscious pain, is mastering your mind, accessing your inner power, and using the power of your mind and mindset. This is critical to you thriving and feeling alive. Mastering your mind in relation to your fibro is the foundation upon which everything else depends, because your mind determines your thoughts that directly impact your feelings, emotions and actions, which shape your reality. Believe me when I say, fibromyalgia is not in the mind, it is very real, but you have to use the power of your mind and conscious thought, to not let it get the better of you.

As previously mentioned, what we focus on expands. This book is focused on replacing the negative and bad in your life, with the positive, happy and good, so you can get a natural high from dopamine, rather than from medications that are not solving the root cause of your pain, but just getting you to rely on unhealthy habits that are a temporary fix. It is about creating a pocket in your mind, where you are as unconscious as possible of your pain, because you make a conscious choice to become unconscious of it, to safeguard yourself against it.

STOP FOCUSING ON THE KRYPTONITE!

If you are in a lot of pain, a fibromyalgia group online or offline may feel supportive; you tell them about your pain, they tell you about theirs, you can relate to one another and understand each other when no one else can, but you are also focusing on that pain; bringing it to the forefront of your mind, and living in your head in your pain. In essence, it perpetuates that feeling of pain. That is why, although I am in online fibromyalgia groups and I deeply value what they do for us, I no longer spend much time in them like I first used to.

Instead of talking about and focusing on your pain, what you should be doing is to separate a section of your mind, where your soul can comfortably live unconscious of your pain. Make this your little pocket of freedom from pain in your mind. You can do this because your mind is not your body; it's separate. Think of your body down below as a vessel, and your mind as the centre of who you are. Think that it does not matter what your body does, because your mind is with you; your mind is who you are and your body is separate. That way you focus less on your body pain and more on you. This is a time when you need to live more in your mind than your body, or more specifically, you need to live in that pocket of conscious thought that is away from your body, that has the right mindset and is unconscious of your pain. I have trained myself to do that and so can you.

Think of being on stage, you have an audience of people called pain watching you, you focus on that pain and feel their negative energy and that affects your performance. You cannot wait for that curtain to come down. You struggle and struggle, and the more you focus on that pain, it's like kryptonite for your soul as it penetrates your being and infiltrates your cells. It's too late, it's spreading like a disease and you feel absolutely powerless; you feel like it's the end. But you see the curtain lever out of the corner of your eye. You stop focusing on the audience of pain, and you turn to view that lever, you see it fully and your eyes zoom in on it. You no longer look at the audience of pain, but you give that lever your full attention, you are drawn to it, and you focus on just that lever, so much so, that the whole room nearly becomes greyed out, and you start walking towards it. You feel compelled to pull that lever down, and that feeling becomes stronger and stronger as you move towards it, with total focus, almost unaware of your surroundings, all you can think about is that lever and the excitement that goes with the anticipation that you can pull it down and be free from your pain. You march; stride; and dive towards it like a soldier on fire that needs immediate water to put out those flames! You grasp that lever with both hands and you pull it firmly down, the red curtain drops and you are finally free from the audience of pain. You feel relieved, and a sense of warmth comes over your body. You love being behind that curtain, because you feel protected in your little cocoon, free of pain and the direct link to that kryptonite. You escape through back stage doors, and when you next emerge on stage, in front of your audience of pain, you make sure you are wearing a full suit of armour, standing proud as your superhero self; unleashed from the chains of your pain; standing strong and in control; with a determination to succeed against whatever the world throws at you, so that the audience of pain cannot set-up that kryptonite to go right through you ever again and you can easily escape behind that curtain, (that pocket of your mind (conscious thought), that is free from conscious pain), whenever you want. Think of it as your suit of mind protection armour when going out in public. So long as no one creates some extra pain to penetrate that armour, you will be okay and set up for battle. And not only that, you can live behind that curtain to stay free and oblivious to pain, whilst projecting yourself to the outside world in your body armour for protection.

So in essence, in your fibro life, you always have your body that is separate from your mind and acts as your physical armour against the world and is what people see. And just like a superhero, you have that warm glowing energy that is your heart; soul; and inner intuition; that bathes your inside cells, makes you aware of your surroundings and is super perceptive; while allowing you to see; sense; and do extraordinary things. And at the same time, you have separated a relatively large section of the upper part of your mind and brain, which has a thick set of red stage curtains firmly around and in front of it. Your unconscious lives there pain free, and pays no mind to the rest of your brain that is conscious of it. It is also where you apply positive self-talk; your antidotes; your authentic self, whilst using mind distractions, engrossment and engagement, to keep your mind free from pain.

Nourish that special pocket of your brain with positivity and an unstoppable attitude. That way you can achieve things you never thought possible whilst having fibromyalgia and this is where the magic takes place of my best-kept secret and of my 21st mindset – more about these later. This is why sometimes meditation, does NOT work for fibromyalgia sufferers, if the meditation requires you to focus on how your body feels and you are in pain, you are focusing on that pain.

This pocket of your mind that is separate to your body, is one technique I use consistently, every day, to give my mind a break from my body pain. In other words, I use the power of my mind to block out the pain. It means I consciously choose to make a pocket of space in my subconscious where I am free of conscious pain. So I am able to be unconscious of my pain, in that pocket of my brain (remember that curtain you are behind), by essentially not thinking about it, keeping the rest of my mind busy and distracted with other things, and thinking about being pain free. It works well if you refrain from verbally talking about fibro as much as possible and from writing about it. In essence, you need to free your mind and life from your conscious pain as much as possible, by freeing your conscious thoughts of it. If something brings me back to 'reality', such as climbing stairs, which makes my legs hurt significantly more than the rest of my body, I then become briefly conscious of my pain again being much worse than the rest of the time. If I mention I have fibro to someone, it helps more than if I say the whole word fibromyalgia, because it is more casual and less like the word to me, and therefore does not instigate the full force of fibromyalgia pain. But to not mention I have it at all, whenever possible, works best. However, if I do something to cause myself greater pain than I would normally experience with my fibromyalgia, such as lift something heavy above shoulder height and hurt my arms in the process, as my inner muscles are weak, this can be felt, as it goes above my threshold pain for this pain free pocket of my brain. In other words, it upsets the equilibrium of my body, and I notice I have hurt myself. And this is the only time I may take painkillers such as Ibuprofen or Paracetamol, not for fibromyalgia that puts my body in a constant state of pain particularly where my legs are joined to my pelvis, but for extra pain on top of it. Currently this does not happen too often and I will only take them as a last resort and buy specific brands that I know don't cause me any side effects, and consume them for the least amount of time possible. I can go for a long time without painkillers and take less now than I used to before I had fibro! The pharmaceutical industry is big business, the more pills you take, the more money they make and therefore it works in their interests if you need one pill to counteract the effects of another. Notice that it's in *their* interests, not yours. If you need one pill, to counteract the effects of another, it can lead to a vicious cycle of pill taking. And all of these side effects can cause more problems than the original problem. I knew someone who was on fibromyalgia medication; they seemed to have swelling due to the medication they were on, which made their overall condition worse. I have family members, who don't have fibro, but seem to exhibit more side effects from some medications, than some of their problems in the first place. I read posts from people in fibromyalgia groups and posts on their timeline, saying they are in excruciating pain and are taking X, Y, Z medication, it never seems to occur to them it could be the medication causing this pain. They say I am taking this now, as that didn't work. I tried this; I tried that. I am on that, I am on this, and often they are bed ridden for hours on end, their body in a consistent flare up. Which is not surprising considering the side effects. The stuff they are taking, to my mind, is lethal for the body. I would rather live with my fibro pain, than take any meds directly for it. I don't want to consistently pump my body full of chemicals that need more chemicals, just imagine what all those chemicals are doing to your body; killing off all the good bacteria in your body, as well as no doubt lowering your immune system, so you get more illnesses and need more pills. Can you see a pattern here? Speaking of good bacteria, I had over 3 years at my day job, with no time off sick, working a 38.5 hour week, which I put down to being helped by the fact I buy good bacteria in liquid form from a homeopath, to support my immune system, before and after an infection. I was also taking some each week for those 3 years to prevent illness. Nowadays, if I feel like I have a slight sore throat, I usually keep some of these good bacteria in stock to keep topped up with good bugs, so my body can defend itself and stand a good chance of not getting ill or it turning into more. Remember, prevention is ALWAYS better than cure. If you do your research, you will discover the bacteria you see in yoghurts in the supermarket are not usually enough in numbers and the capsules you buy in health shops, often the bacteria die off before they reach your mouth. So a little tip to help your fibromyalgia and your immune system, buy good bacteria in liquid form at the very least, whenever you have taken antibiotics. Antibiotics kill off the good bacteria in your gut, as well as the bad, so if you don't replenish the good bacteria after you stop taking the antibiotics, you will have a swamp full of bad bacteria thriving in your gut, with no defence to stop them causing you more infections and illnesses. So if you find you get one illness after another, this is probably why, you are all out of good bacteria. And remember, I am talking about alternative therapies to the doctor's pills, which most doctors I find, do not support. If it is not conventional pills, they don't want to know or hear about it and they won't support it or believe in it. I know homeopathy works for me and I have found other natural products for conditions that I would have had to take pills for, or continue on prescribed medications forever.

KEY POINTS TO REMEMBER

The most crucial thing to managing your fibromyalgia and decreasing your conscious pain, is mastering your mind.

Sometimes fibromyalgia groups both online and offline can be and feel supportive, but they can also keep your head in your pain.

What we focus on expands. If we talk about being in pain, and think about it, we will experience more of it, as we are bringing it to our conscious thoughts.

Separate a section of your mind, away from your pain, a large section, where your soul can comfortably live behind your curtain of armour to protect you. This is your little pocket of freedom from pain in your mind.

PART 4
HOW TO MASTER YOUR ENVIRONMENTS
TO AVOID AN EXPLOSION!

CHAPTER 12
THE VOLCANO EFFECT

Remember that quote:

"Feeling good is the antidote to feeling bad. Feeling pleasure is the antidote to feeling pain. Feeling happy is the antidote to feeling sad. Feeling safe; loved and having faith, is the antidote to feeling fear."

If you strive to obtain these antidotes and keep your core being and body in these positive feeling states, your body will reward you with less pain. If not, it will be like hot liquid building up inside of you, attracting bits of hard rock along the way, gaining momentum. The more it is subjected to the wrong things the more forceful it will push against your insides, until it keeps building up and building up, and finally flares up and explodes with the pressure, bubbling over like hot lava, leaving a trail of destruction in its path. It's not until you can control these symptoms of bad feelings, before they get out of hand, that you will be able to manage your fibro pain to a degree that you can cope with in everyday life and lead a relatively 'normal' existence.

So how do you get from where you are now, to having all of those feelings, to make your body be in the best possible state, to have the least amount of pain? We have to address both your internal and external environments and make improvements in each area of them because oftentimes, your internal and external environments directly impact each other. How we live both internally and externally is key to managing fibromyalgia.

Your internal environment includes:

- ✓ Your body.
- ✓ Foods you consume.
- ✓ Medications you take.
- ✓ Your mind.
- ✓ Thoughts.
- ✓ Feelings.
- ✓ Emotions.
- ✓ Spirit/Soul.
- ✓ Relationship with yourself.
- ✓ Intuition.
- ✓ Your mission.

Your external environment includes:

- ✓ Relationships with others.
- ✓ Home layout and design.
- ✓ Lifestyle
- ✓ Clothes.
- ✓ Finances.
- ✓ Career/Job.
- ✓ Hobbies.

We have already addressed many of these environments in previous chapters; such as the relationship you have with yourself and others; the medications you take, which we will be discussing more in the next chapter; your mindset, and the correlation between your mind, body, thoughts, feelings, and emotions. We also discussed about how to use my Embrace Your Quirky philosophy to nourish your soul, and that you should follow your heart as it will help increase your energy and reduce your pain. We discussed how your pain gives you superhero abilities, and heightens your sensitivity to situations that are no good for you, so you should listen to your intuition to keep pain at bay. In the chapters that follow, we will address your other environments.

KEY POINTS TO REMEMBER

It's not until you can control symptoms of bad feelings, before they get out of hand, that you will be able to manage your fibro pain to a degree that you can cope with it in everyday life and lead a relatively 'normal' existence.

How we live both internally and externally is key to managing fibromyalgia.

Your internal and external environments directly impact each other.

We have to address both your internal and external environments and make improvements in each area of them to reduce your fibro pain.

CHAPTER 13
FOODS TO EAT AND FOODS
TO AVOID

What foods we put into our body impacts our pain and health. When you put a food into your body that depletes your energy – which is what taking refined sugars does to me – you don't feel like doing much; talking to anyone, and you just want to go to bed and sleep. This will affect your relationship with yourself, as you will feel depressed that you are spending so much time sleeping and have a lack of energy; with your friends, as you will be too tired to see them and may have to cancel plans with them; with your partner, as you will not feel up to doing much with them, you may not even feel like talking, you may just need some time to sleep instead of spending time with them and they may feel rejected. In such circumstances, it is essential you do something about your situation as you cannot continue with this quality of life, and you must communicate effectively your current situation to those it may impact.

I first discovered I had an allergy to sugar at only 15 years of age. People believe sugar gives them energy, but in my case it doesn't. The homeopath said a lot of people have an allergy to sugar, they just don't realise it, and that is what makes them feel tired. I remember eating an apple pie and that made my tummy hurt and sting. The homeopath had helped my mum to be less ill with her ME, so I trusted him. Still, I was nearly a chocoholic back then, and I just had to try every new chocolate bar that came out. I especially loved it when they added an orange or mint flavour to a core line, to make it that bit different. So I never gave sugar up, I did not listen. By age 19, I got so ill from eating sugar, that I was doing a part-time job for only 3 hours a day, 5 days a week, and I did my usual bit of food shopping on the way home, whilst feeling dizzy, having tummy pain, and my eyebrows were heavy in my head. When I got home I went to bed at some ridiculous early hour. Sugar is the death of my energy and my quality of life and by 19 years of age, I realised I could not go on like this. Only 15 hours of work a week and feeling ill and going home to sleep, was not my idea of enjoying life or of feeling alive. So I went back to the homeopath and I finally took my sugar allergy diagnosis seriously, and decided it was no longer worth me having headaches and feeling tired after just 3 hours of work and gave it up, and I have not looked back since. So let me ask you a question. Do you eat sugar and are you constantly feeling tired? You could argue it's your fibro, but what is causing your fibro tiredness? Is it sugar and you just don't realise it? Or does your fear of giving up sugar mean you don't even want to think about it and you would rather remain oblivious to that real answer? Try cutting out all refined sugars, this includes dextrose; sucrose; glucose; do it for at least a month and see how you feel. Try it for up to 3 months and see what a difference it makes to your life and wellbeing.

So what foods do I avoid and consume? I do not drink any alcohol; I gave that up when I gave up sugar at 19. I don't drink any caffeine or smoke anything, and I have never tried recreational drugs or a cigarette.

My Allergies:

- Sugar: All refined sugars including glucose, sucrose, and dextrose. I can still have natural sugars in fruit juices, so long as there is no added sugar.

- Wheat.

- MSG (Monosodium Glutamate derived from wheat).

- Spelt (Alternative to wheat).

- Strawberries, Raspberries and Blueberries – Although I can have a few of those, whereas my other allergies I have to completely avoid. Strawberries are definitely the worst. A couple of years ago I ate two small clotted cream size pots of them and the next evening my bottom lip swelled up like the professor's in the film Nutty Professor. Sometimes my allergies give me an instant reaction, sometimes a delayed reaction.

My Intolerances:

- Gluten.

- Yeast. It causes candida overgrowth in the gut, so does anything that can be classed as a mouldy product such as mushrooms, grapes, and cheeses, or fermented, such as yogurts and oyster sauce, so I don't eat any of those. I slipped up by mistake in 2017 and ate one pot of natural lactose free yoghurt, forgetting it was fermented, and boy did I have tummy ache afterwards. Even though there are numerous articles saying to eat this stuff, it's not good in this way.

- Lactose. Which is a sugar found in milk.

- Dairy.

I believe not consuming any of these foods and food ingredients in my diet cause me to have less pain and more energy. From the research I have done, wheat is very bad for fibromyalgia pain and should be cut out of your diet, so should MSG that is derived from wheat and often found in flavoured crisps. Gluten is another I would definitely recommend cutting out. Sugar is no good either, so cut it. Stop drinking alcohol, it's full of sugar and your liver has to work harder to get rid of those extra toxins, and your body is already under strain from having fibromyalgia, it does not need any more.

Berries are a good source of antioxidants for the body. Try eliminating all of the others foods one-by-one to see if your pain decreases and if you get rashes or swelling from eating berries, you will need to eliminate them too.

Monitor your carb intake to see if certain carbs make you feel tired and in pain, so you can adjust your diet to have less of those, or cut them completely if you are able to. If you have low blood sugar, you will usually always need to have some carbs, so consult a doctor or qualified nutritionist about this. Some carbs such as plain ready salted crisps give me energy. I get low blood sugar, so I tend to eat some carbs throughout the day to stay energised

What I am about to share with you is something you need to incorporate into your weekly diet. If you don't pay attention to anything else I tell you about what to eat and what not to eat, please, please, pay attention to this. An essential food I added to my diet in 2014 was mackerel, for the high level of omega 3s it contains. The results are astonishing; it feels like the insides of my legs are being bathed in oil. I love sea bass, but the omega 3s are not a high enough dosage to decrease my pain, so although I don't like the taste of mackerel that much, the benefits of taking it far outweigh the taste, as it significantly decreases my leg pain so much so, that it's less painful to walk up hills, and I can jog or even run up the road a bit. To improve its taste, some of the herbs I add to it are rosemary or thyme, sometimes I add crushed chillies depending on how my digestive system is feeling, and at other times I use lemon and black pepper or black pepper on its own. I will add mixed herbs to vegetables for seasoning. If eating out in a restaurant, I will ask for the food to be plain, without any sauces, and change it according to my dietary needs. If I haven't eaten mackerel in about 3 days, by the 4th day my legs return to feeling like they have been run over by a bus. So make sure you add mackerel to your diet in it's natural form and not smoked. You need to ideally eat it every day, and never let more than 3 days pass without consuming it, as it is essential for decreasing pain – even pain in the abdomen it can help decrease! Just be aware that the natural fat content is high but it's good fats your body needs. I don't take CBD oil and I never would. Mackerel is the natural wonder food you need to eat daily to bathe your inner body in oil to ease your pain. Eat Mackerel in conjunction with everything else I explain to eat and drink, and eliminate all those foods and drinks I say are bad for fibromyalgia. Do as I do in this book, and you should feel so much better, and in less pain.

Green leafy vegetables are great to eat and this includes spinach. Whenever I eat spinach I feel so much better and more vibrant. Broccoli is great too and you can eat both of these raw or cooked, but raw maintains more of its nutrients and so it is more beneficial. The same homeopath told me that tomatoes are not good for the stomach because they act like Aspirin. I find cherry tomatoes to be okay for my tummy, but any others hurt my tummy, as do apples, although I can drink apple juice, so I haven't eaten apples or 'normal' tomatoes for years. It is important when you eat and drink, to note how your body reacts to what you consume. Really concentrate on how your body feels and whether a food sets off a fibro flare, a growling in your tummy, a stinging sensation, a gurgling noise, or other. If any of this happens repeatedly with certain foods or drink, you know to start eliminating them from your diet completely.

Fresh fruit and veg should make up a huge part of your diet. For a snack try eating pressed fruit bars, or pressed fruit and nut bars with nothing added, such as Naked bars, providing you can eat nuts and they don't cause a problem with your digestion. They have a range of Naked Bars with different ingredients in them and as I avoid eating all mouldy products and I discovered from my research that included grapes, I don't usually eat anything with grapes in them, and this includes raisins that are dried grapes, so I don't buy Naked bars that contain those. Again, I am not saying you will like them, I am just saying what I like to eat as a healthy snack. You can also get bars from other manufacturers that just have pressed fruit and no nuts, which I also eat.

Besides eating fruits like peaches and nectarines, other snacks I eat are plain crisps, not flavoured, as they have MSG in them, and I also eat lentil crisps that are gluten free. I try to find crisps with high oleic sunflower oil in them and sea salt, which is better for my body.

Nearly all breakfast cereals have sugar as part of their ingredients. Remember I said it's important to eliminate sugar from your diet, so from now on you will need to look at the ingredients of everything you buy and eat. I often eat puffed rice for breakfast with unsweetened soya milk. This puffed rice is natural with nothing added and found in the 'gluten free' section of one of my local supermarkets, they also sell it at my local independent health store too. Just because something is gluten free, does not mean it is sugar free. In fact many gluten free products do contain sugar, so it's important to always read the ingredients. Other times I have a natural pressed fruit and nut bar for breakfast. If I go away on holiday, I either take my soya milk and cereal with me in my case, or I will eat fish and fruit for breakfast if the hotel has that on its menu. I phone up to discuss this with the hotel before I go. Toast is not to be eaten as it's made from wheat, and wheat is something you should stop eating forever with fibromyalgia.

It is well known that white meats are healthier for you than red. I don't eat lamb or beef and I also don't eat pork – even though some people see that as white meat, it's very fatty! So my diet is either chicken or fish, with vegetables or salad, and sometimes a jacket potato, or plain rice or rice noodles. The simple rule is to keep it plain and as natural as possible, even when eating out! If you look at a restaurant menu and there is a meal you would be able to eat, if it didn't come with an ingredient you cannot eat, ask the staff if they can make adjustments for you. I do this regularly. So I can't eat a chicken breast burger in a bun, but I can eat the plain chicken breast without the bun and sauces, which is what I ask for, providing it does not have any allergens added to the burger, such as dextrose, which is a sugar, and I have to ask them to check to ensure it does not have this also.

A fellow entrepreneur who used to be bed ridden with fibromyalgia confirmed that what we put into our body directly affects our pain. He said corn was another food he had to cut from his diet. I know sometimes it affects my digestion so try reducing your consumption of that or cut it out completely.

My former business advisor used to be a nutrition specialist and said magnesium is great for alleviating fibromyalgia pain, although I got a supplement of this with calcium and it did not seem to make any difference to me. So try it and see if it works for you.

You need to experiment and find out what works for you, but please don't be ignorant to what is actually hurting you. If you are reaching for that cream cake and you know it is going to give you pain, give it up! Do you want to change your life or not? Or do you want to tell your mind, it's fine, tomorrow I will give it up? Remember, your objective is to reduce your pain as much as possible, and one part of this is paying attention to your diet; the foods you eat; what you are putting into your mouth, as it directly affects your body. Your body is part of your internal environment. In order to reduce your fibromyalgia pain, you need to assess both your internal and external environment and get them into the best possible state to reduce your pain and help you to lead a better quality of life.

KEY POINTS TO REMEMBER

What foods we put into our body impacts our pain and health.

When you put a food into your body that depletes your energy you don't feel like doing much; talking to anyone, and you just want to go to bed and sleep. This will affect your relationship with yourself and others.

A lot of people have an allergy to sugar, they just don't realise it, and that is what makes them feel tired.

Cut out these foods from your diet; dairy; yeast; refined sugars, including alcohol; wheat; MSG and gluten; fermented and mouldy products, to reduce your pain.

Add green leafy vegetables such as spinach and broccoli to your diet.

Make fruit and veg a main part of your diet.

This is super important advice. Make sure you listen to this if nothing else, as it can significantly reduce your pain. Eat mackerel <u>daily</u> for omega 3s to reduce your pain. This works

really well as it feels like the insides of your legs are being bathed in oil, making it far easier to walk, jog, or even run.

The simple rule is to keep food as plain and as natural as possible, even when eating out! If you look at a restaurant menu and there is a meal you would be able to eat, if it didn't come with an ingredient you cannot eat, ask the staff if they can make adjustments for you.

Pay attention to how your body feels when consuming different foods.

Give up foods that you know cause you pain.

CHAPTER 14
NATURAL REMEDIES

I mentioned in a previous chapter you should take a liquid form of good bacteria after antibiotics and to maintain a healthy immune system to prevent illness. I take something call Hylak, but my bacteria strain mixture is suitable for my body because I had the homeopath assess me first. Everybody's body is different, so I would suggest seeing a qualified homeopath first, to find out what works well for your body. Be careful to get a reputable one.

From my own research of fibromyalgia, it's known to be an auto-immune disease as I mentioned in an earlier chapter, and you can get other illnesses because of it. I have had two other major health problems in my life that while not necessarily directly related to fibro, I would like to share with you, in case you find yourself in a similar situation. If I can help just one more person to live a better quality of life by reading what helped me in these situations, then I will be happy.

If you knew me, you would know I have a natural abundance of energy, which is very different to most fibro sufferers, but at one particular point in my life several years ago, I knew something was deeply wrong, I felt like an 80 year old woman inside my being. I had to go to the doctor and have a blood test to determine what was wrong. Even as I write this I feel faint at the thought of it, needles and blood being taken from me, usually results in me almost passing out. And I almost pass out seeing anything like that with anyone else. When my mum had a major operation, I went a very pale colour at the sight of tubes linked up to her and the nurses were more concerned about me falling on the floor than my mum's post-op condition and I had to leave the ward to sit down in the corridor for a bit. So you know, for me to go to the doctors, with the knowledge I would most likely have to have a blood test, meant it was a last resort for me to do that and my condition was quite serious. The blood test results showed I had the beginnings of hypothyroidism. I basically had a lack of the Thyroxin hormone in my body. This hormone is essential to keep the thyroid working properly, if it doesn't work, it can be fatal. The doctor said I would need another blood test in 3 months time and if that showed I fell below a certain number on the TSH scale, I would then need to be on hormone replacement therapy for the rest of my life. This would mean regular blood tests to get the right hormone level and to monitor it. Me, blood tests!! Did I mention I hate them? This was enough to spur me on to take my life into my own hands and to research how to get Thyroxin, naturally. After two weeks of re-search, I discovered iodine was key to increasing Thyroxin levels in the blood and that you need a certain amount each day to func-tion properly. Iodine is in seaweed, otherwise known as kelp, and you can buy kelp in capsule form to take daily to get that iodine fix. Although having multiple food allergies and intolerances is a bless-ing in disguise as many of those foods seem to be no good for fibro and increase pain, it makes buying natural supplements more ex-pensive, because I cannot have just have any bottle of kelp from mainstream health shops, as these are packed with additives and not pure. The objective is to get as much natural kelp in my body as I need, not mixed with other stuff that isn't any good for me and may cause my body to flare up. So I went to my local independent health shop. Remember when I said to believe everything happens for a reason, well what are the odds of what I am about to tell you, happening? The woman who at that time owned the shop, I ex-plained to her about my research and she said her husband was rushed into hospital with hypothyroidism and is on hormone re-placement therapy for the rest of his life. She had a bottle of <u>Viridi-an Kelp</u>, that was just seaweed in a cellulose capsule, and nothing else, and she said in a super serious tone of voice, that if this works, you will HAVE to take these for the rest of your life, daily, in place of hormone replacement therapy, and made sure I under-stood this. I nodded and understood. She added that once you start taking hormone replacement therapy, you cannot then use the kelp; you have to use it instead of the therapy, before you ever have to go on it. I took it consistently for the remaining duration of those 3 months and when it came to my next blood test, guess what? That's right, my TSH levels were almost smack bang in the middle of the scale, where they should be. So I knew I had my solu-tion for life. At a later appointment, I told the doctor I have iodine in the form of kelp and explained what happened, she said my re-sults must have been a blip before, and that they used to recom-mend iodine, but no longer did. I wonder why that could be, Oooohhh let me think, oh yes, more pills would be needed if I had not made my discovery, more money for the pharmaceutical in-dustry, so can you see how this pattern keeps cropping up and smacks you right in the face!! Do you see it? Your body environ-ment should be natural, so it makes sense to treat it with natural products, not pump it with one pill after another on a regular ba-sis. Ask yourself, are my pills really reducing my pain? Are they causing me any more problems? And then ask yourself, what am I going to do about it? I still use these kelp capsules to this day. In fact I used to take 2, which gave me 840ug of iodine a day, but something strange happened to me in 2016 and I began to feel like an old woman again, so I upped my dose to 3 a day, a total of 1260ug in iodine content, as they were 420ug each in iodine con-tent, and that solved the problem. It was slightly over the recom-mended dose I had read about, which was 1000ug (otherwise

known as 1000mcg – micrograms) at the time, some websites recommend far less these days, but I still stick to the same as I know
these work for me; I had the blood test which proved to me that
800ug was the right dosage for me at the time, or almost, as it was
'nearly' smack bang in the middle of the scale where is should have
been; and that amount keeps my energy levels at the right level for
me. It's interesting for me to observe the differences between a
blog or website based on taking medicinal pills which promotes all
the risks involved with taking kelp to help with thyroid and advis-
es against it, such as this one http://www.btf-
thyroid.org/projects/iodine/249-iodine-faq to a blog and website
about using natural products and all the immense benefits of taking kelp including helping with thyroid function, such as this one
https://www.livestrong.com/article/507585-the-dosage-of-kelp-
for-thyroid-function/ Kelp hasn't made me lose weight, which it
suggests in this post it can do, and I put a bit on since being redundant as I don't walk to work every day and back again, which took
20-25 minutes each way, 5 days a week, but I do some walking at
least 3 times a week, and I tend to stay at a relatively stable weight
since then which fluctuates by a few pounds depending on what I
eat that day. Walking is very good for helping to stop hip pain, as
well as some exercises I got from a physiotherapist via my doctor.
So it's worth going to see a qualified physiotherapist to get advice
about what exercises to do to help with your specific fibromyalgia
needs. Get a physiotherapist that will encourage you to do some
exercises, and allow you to adapt the exercises to your own specific fibro pain thresholds. Remember, you should expect to be in a
bit more pain initially as you start to slowly work parts of the body
and muscles that you may not usually use, or not use that often,
but think of the gain you will have as your body should become far
more flexible, and in less pain in the long run - if you eat mackerel
too, and get the rest of your food intake correct as described in this

book and wear the correct footwear as I describe in this book, and get the correct bed as I describe in this book, and get the correct environment as described in this book, and don't focus on your pain. This book needs to be used as a complete system to reduce your overall pain, as everything I explain in these 25 aspects of your life, throughout the chapters in this book, have a knock on effect with other areas of your life. Even if you have a positive mindset, if you are putting foods in your body that are harmful to it, your body flares up in pain as a result. So you have to eliminate and limit, as many of those pain triggers as possible, in those multiple aspects of your life, to reduce your pain. Think of your fibromyalgia as soaking up all different types of pain in your life like a sponge, and you feel that pain 10 times more than the average person. In this way it's your superpower, as it alerts you to all of those areas of pain in your life. Think of it like having X-ray vision, it shows you the pain areas of your life, that you may otherwise have not noticed. In this way your fibro is actually working for you, not against you, if only you would allow yourself to think that way, instead of all the negativity surrounding fibro and programmed into your mind through conditioning.

Viridian made the capsules smaller and now you need to buy more to get the same dosage, so as I write this book I take 6 Viridian Kelp capsules which are 286mg of kelp in each capsule, which gives me 200ug of iodine in each, a total of 1200ug (ug is otherwise known as mcg (micrograms) each day). I did try to have just 1000ug with a total of 5 capsules and that didn't work for me. I started to feel my energy levels were never quite right and to feel older inside again. Like I said before, I am no medical professional so you should always consult one of those, and you should consult a qualified homeopath or healthcare practitioner to get the kelp and iodine dosage that's right for you. Incidentally, I found that the iodine in kelp helps to counteract the effects of the fluoride poisoning problem with fluoride toothpastes. If you have never heard of this problem before and you thought your toothpaste was just this sweet and innocent little blob you put into your mouth to clean your teeth and make them shiny and white, think again! If you Google 'fluoride poisoning', you will soon discover that fluoride is toxic. There are a couple of good articles about this on the website www.naturalnews.com. One is titled, "Fluoride depletes iodine in the body, causing hypothyroidism and immune deficiency", in this article, written by Marianne Leigh, she explains that:

"Fluoride is getting a lot of bad press these days, and for good reason: it is a toxic molecule that wreaks extensive, often irreversible, havoc on the body. The thyroid is particularly affected by fluoride exposure because its store of iodine is depleted. Iodine deficiency depresses the thyroid's metabolic and immune functions, resulting in hypothyroidism and lowered immunity."

In this article she goes on to explain how this happens and some of the side effects:

"Lack of iodine shuts down production of thyroxine, the thyroid prohormone that controls metabolism, and, in one way or another, impacts every aspect of health. The resulting hypothyroidism causes weight gain, cold intolerance, dry and prematurely aged skin, depression, constipation, hair loss, memory loss, irritability, increased cholesterol levels, heart disease and loss of libido."

Does this sound familiar? Do any of these symptoms resemble those of fibromyalgia?

In another article on the same website, www.naturalnews.com, written by Barbara L. Minton, titled, "Hypothyroidism Reaches Epidemic Proportions, Causing Fatigue And Weight Gain", Barbara Explains:

"Hypothyroidism is behind many disease states: Hypothyroidism is signaled by fatigue and loss of energy. People with the disease don't have any sparkle in the morning, and as the day goes on they find themselves falling asleep sitting in meetings or while driving on the highway, reading or watching TV. The only time they feel energized is from continuous movement, such as jogging or doing housework. As soon as the task is completed and they sit down, chances are good they will start to nod off. Yet while they are fatigued, low thyroid people are often hyperactive at the same time. Barbara goes onto say, "People with low thyroid exhibit many of the characteristics that are blamed on aging, with difficulty concentrating being the most blatant. They tend to flit from task to task and often accomplish little they set out to do. They can find themselves standing in front of an open refrigerator, unable to remember what they are looking for. They may have difficulty reading, needing to read sentences again because their mind wandered off the first time."

Sound familiar? What is even more surprising and stoked my curiosity is a section of the article that states:

"Epidemiological studies of radiation downwinders show many of the symptoms of hypothyroidism including chronic fatigue syndrome and fibromyalgia. According to Dr. Peat, fibromyalgia is a combination of edema, inflammation and low blood sugar, all symptoms of hypothyroidism. He too believes that radiation is a major culprit in the hypothyroid epidemic."

Gives food for thought doesn't it? Unfortunately, as of yet, I have not found a suitable non-fluoride toothpaste alternative for my sensitive teeth and gum receding problem! One which will not leave my mouth and the side of my face in constant debilitating pain, but I have my kelp as my weapon in the fight against it! Unfortunately, if you went to your doctor for fluoride poisoning, you would most probably be given some sort of weird look to say the least! I haven't tried it, but I know whenever I bring up natural so-lutions, my doctor does not agree with them! Some locum doctors have had a better attitude. So I try not to see my doctor for such things if I can help it and treat myself as much as possible.

Some people with fibromyalgia report not having any improve-ment from the medication they have been prescribed. Ask your-self, is your fibromyalgia pain decreased by your medication and not causing you any side effects? Think back to before you started taking any medications and if you have developed any further health problems since then? Fibromyalgia can cause swelling and tingling and numbness in areas of your body such as your hands, but so can other illnesses and some medications. You need to work out if it is the fibromyalgia causing it, or something else, or the medications you are taking. Because I don't take meds for fibro, I know my pain is not from meds, it is either from my fibro or an-other underlying health condition. It could be I have hurt my neck but because the pain is extra to my usual neck pain and is travel-ling down my shoulders and up and down my arms into my wrists, hands and fingers, I know the cause is not my fibro.

I am no doctor or medical health professional, and these are my own opinions and thoughts, so please consult one of those before doing anything with any medications you are taking. Pills have their place and can save lives. If you are under medical supervision and need a prescribed pill to save your life, or for a life threatening condition, then of course I believe you should take it and I would tell you to, life is the most precious gift and we have to do whatev-er it takes to save it. I would also encourage researching about al-ternative medicines if pills are failing. My mum's life has been saved by conventional treatment and follow up medications. If you are taking tablets that are not causing you any side effects or dam-age to your body short-term or long-term, and there are no natural alternatives that will be as effective, then there is no reason not to take them if you want to. You just have to realise that the pharmaceutical industry is worth big bucks, so it pays to get you to take medications for life or as long as possible, and often these pills are not curing the root cause of the problem. I believe that sometimes there are natural alternatives to taking pills that are not working for you and actually causing your body more harm than good. I even buy a <u>Sea Kelp shampoo</u> for my hair, which appears to be free of added wheat, to prevent an itchy scalp that I used to get from using conventional shampoos in the past. I get it from a health shop and the brand is called "Jason". It is free from parabens, sulfates, phthalates, petrolatum, and artificial colours. You have to take each situation as it comes but be prepared to seek out as many natural solutions as possible and keep an open mind.

NOW I AM GOING TO SHOCK YOU!

So now I am going to shock you and tell you about a time I was 'forced' to be on 8 tablets a day, yes, I did say 8 a day!!! You may be able to guess the outcome of what I am about to tell you, but I am just going to go right ahead and tell you anyhow. It was December 2013, and I had been off work sick for a couple of days with a Gastroenteritis infection. After 48 hours had passed I was supposed to be non-contagious. A few days later I went to a work meeting in the city of Bristol, in the UK. During that train journey my tummy did not feel right and it hurt. But it was not until after I had eaten lunch that the pain really set in. It resulted in me not being able to stand up to even go to the toilet and an ambulance was called. The doctor saw me at the hospital and diagnosed me with gastritis as a result of my previous gastroenteritis. It meant I would need to get a prescription of a few different tablets to solve the problem. With a further diagnosis of the lining of my stomach being damaged, I was off for a total of 4 weeks from my work, or day job, as I liked to call it. I went back to work too soon because my boss at that time was putting pressure on me, and I got a respiratory infection, lost my voice, and had to have another week off. After being back at work since January 21st, around March/April time, I was concerned I was still on 8 tablets a day and getting pain in my chest when I ate, and food regurgitation in my throat, despite the fact I had stopped drinking peppermint tea, as I got told by the doctor that it would make my type of acid reflux worse. On his advice, I had tried to reduce the tablets, but couldn't as my symptoms got worse, and to top it off, I had developed a highly visible red rash on my neck as a side effect from the tablets I was taking. I could not go on like it. So I saw the doctor and explained all this, and guess what? I was told he could not do anything else for me. This was as good as it gets. Was I prepared to accept that for the rest of my life, forever? No. Note this, how we get treated, is how we 'accept' to be treated. Thank goodness I have a brain and can think for myself. I researched online and found out that as some people get older, their digestive enzymes in their body stop working and I would need a supplement that contained these enzymes that my body lacked. So I went to a local health shop and tried a digestive tea along with a small bottle of <u>Viridian Digestive Aid</u> enzymes (the same company who made the kelp I take), and although I noticed it helped ease my problem, it did not solve the problem, so I went to see a nutritionist, paid for a consultation and a month's supply of a tincture to solve my problem and come off the tablets. This had a positive impact, but did not solve the problem. So I took some of the ingredients in the tincture that I thought helped me, Ginger, Liquorice and Chamomile, and got each of these in teabag form, <u>Pukka Three Ginger</u> and <u>Twinings Liquorice</u> and <u>Chamomile</u>. I am not telling you Viridian products or these brands of tea will work for you, I am just telling you exactly what I use to help me. And when I combined these teabags, with taking those <u>Viridian Digestive Aid</u> digestive enzymes twice a day, the difference was remarkable, but something still wasn't quite right. The enzymes I decided were not working like they should be, so instead of taking one twice a day, I took two in the morning before food, and that stopped the problem and I became pill free. No more medications from the doctor for me. I still take two of these digestive enzymes every morning for the rest of my life, in place of those tablets from the doctor, and I increase it to 3 upon occasions where I have eaten something different that has caused my body to react with a new temporary digestive problem. I also continue to regularly drink the teas, particularly ginger, as it is so good for digestion and if my tummy starts feeling in pain and out of sorts, it is often because I have not had a cup of those teas for a while and they can be good for calming the tummy when feeling anxious too. So you see, pills can cause further problems and do not solve the root cause of the problem. But we have the ability to think for ourselves, to find new ways of doing things, to go our own way in life and play by our rules, this is why a rockstar attitude and mindset is essential to combatting fibromyalgia pain.

If I have a lot of acute pain in my neck or arms as opposed to my usual pain, I sometimes use <u>Bell's Muscle Rub</u>, which is used to relieve pain in aching joints and muscles, instead of taking painkillers, and it works really well, but a lot of the time I don't just use a little bit, I plaster it all over the affected area, so from the pain point in the top right of my right arm, up my right shoulder, all around my neck, and down the left shoulder and over the pain point in my left arm. This is not what is says to do on the packaging and it does give a burning sensation, so the more you use, the more you will find it creates a burning sensation but I find this really relieves the pain and is quite bliss as it covers the whole area of acute pain. It's for this reason and the fact that it is a gel that can get on your clothes and make a mess, that I apply it while wearing PJs. It has some natural ingredients such as Sweet Birch Oil, Cajuput Oil and Eucalyptus Oil, but it also comes with a warning not to take it if you are allergic to any of the ingredients or painkillers such as Aspirin, Ibuprofen or other NSAIDs. My mum also introduced me to another gel that is for muscles and joints and advertised as helping with fibro pain. It is called Advance 7; Soothing Massage Gel, by Aquil Laboratory, and although not all of its ingredients are 100% natural, it comes with 7 that are; Green Clay, Harpagophytum Horsetail, Essential Oils Of Peppermint, Rosemary, Cajeput and Thyme! This also gives a burning sensation, and although I haven't used it that often, I do find it helps! So always look for legitimate alternative products for pain relief. I am not saying these will work for you, I am just saying what works for me.

I find wheat bags that you put in the microwave are also useful for reducing inflammation and pain, as is a hot shower. A Jacuzzi is soothing and although I can't swim, I have been told by a medical professional that swimming is good for easing fibro pain. But what works best of all is prevention, rather than cure. So for example, I know that crouching down will cause my legs to badly hurt, so I avoid doing this as much as possible and kneeling down is a big no, no, as I once did that and had pain in my knees for 2 or 3 consecutive days, which felt like I was still in that crouching position putting my weight on them. I also try not to lift above shoulder height as much as possible, because it can set off spasms in my arms. Having said this, I do know that if you don't use muscles, you can lose the use of them, and that I need to do some exercise to prevent my pain from getting worse in certain areas of my body as I need them to be strong, not weak! So I try to do a few exercises each morning on an exercise mat for my back, neck, thighs, core and tummy. I also do some dance moves and jigging on the spot most days – even if they are done sat on a chair! I will push myself to do some things so my muscles don't seize up! And this is very important because if I don't do 10 press-ups for my back, my back is in far more pain for most of the day and if I don't do neck exercises, I become restricted in neck movements. So I would not say to never use a part of your body, and that even if you are in pain, you need to try to exercise your body and the many parts of it in some way to keep it strong!

So always be your own superhero where your health is concerned and rescue yourself from pain as much as possible. Use your superhero senses to find out what feels good and right to you and for you. After all, the most precious life in your hands is your own, and that is the one that should always be a top priority to save from pain, and from external sources that may harm your internal environment. Be confident that you know what's best for you and ensure your internal environment is one in which you don't just survive, but thrive and come alive!

KEY POINTS TO REMEMBER

I don't take any prescribed medication for fibromyalgia.

The pharmaceutical industry is big business, so it's in their interests for you to be prescribed pills, but are they working for you?

You often need to take a pill to counteract the affects of another. This can lead to a vicious pill taking cycle.

Sometimes there are natural alternatives to taking pills that are not working for you and actually causing your body more harm than good.

We have the ability to think for ourselves, to find new ways of doing things, to go our own way in life and play by our own rules.

You can get certain muscle rubs in the form of gels to help relieve your pain.

Wheat bags and a hot shower are good for reducing inflammation and pain.

A Jacuzzi is good for soothing pain.

Pain prevention is better than cure.

Although exercise can hurt you and you can avoid doing moves that you know will hurt you, you should still exercise every part of your body to prevent your muscles from stopping working, even if it means experiencing some pain. Consult a qualified physiotherapist to get a list of exercises that will help with your specific fibro pain needs.

Based on my own knowledge and experience of what works for me, if you have a low TSH (Thyroxin) level, which you would find out from a blood test with your doctor, take 1000ug (otherwise known as 1000mcg – micrograms) of iodine EVERY single day, in the morning before food, in the form of additive free kelp to prevent getting hypothyroidism, BEFORE you have to go on hormone replacement therapy for the rest of your life. This also helps to counteract the effects of fluoride poisoning. Consult a qualified homeopath or other healthcare professional to get the dosage right for you and listen to your own inner being and body, to observe how your body takes to it. I take more than 1000ug a day, even though many articles advise taking less, because from my own research years ago, 1000ug was the daily recommended amount back then, and it stops me feeling like an old woman inside and from lacking in my usual energy. Make sure it's the purest form of kelp you can get. I take pure kelp in a vegetarian cellulose capsule in a base of Organic Alfalfa. It's suitable for vegans and is free from gluten, wheat, lactose, added sugar, salt, yeast, preservatives or artificial colourings. Non-irradiated. Against animal testing. From a company called <u>Viridian</u>. Who currently specify not to use it during pregnancy or lactation unless recommended by a healthcare practitioner. Always read the labels of any natural remedy carefully, just like you should be doing with any medicines you take from the doctor. Remember, many doctors will advise you not to take iodine or kelp, and I started to take kelp before I would be diagnosed with full-blown hypothyroidism, when my own doctor told me I had the beginnings of it; and after 2 weeks of doing my own personal research about iodine and kelp.

In my experience, if your digestive system is not working and you are getting chest pain when you eat and acid reflux and regurgitation, stop drinking peppermint tea and take digestive enzymes, 2 a day, in the morning, for the rest of your life, before food. If eating something spicy or anything that upsets your tummy balance, take an extra enzyme and reduce or eliminate that food from your diet. I use <u>Viridian High Potency Digestive Aid.</u>

For easing digestion and to keep the tummy calm and in less pain, drink <u>Pukka Three Ginger</u> and <u>Twinings Liquorice</u>, and <u>Chamomile herbal teas.</u>

CHAPTER 15
TOO CLOTHES FOR COMFORT

Your clothes can hurt you! This is one thing you won't hear very often, but it's true. Whilst the clothes you wear are not physically punching you, they may still be leaving red marks and bruises, and causing you pain. I find when I layer up in colder weather, and I have one top on top of another, this can cause me to have red marks at my elbow joints and sometimes it causes me to bruise and pumps out pain. So whilst I am trying to look good and keep warm, I am also hurting. This is something you have to accept comes with the fibro bundle, or you wear looser fitting clothing.

I already mentioned at the beginning of this book, that if you suffer with feet swelling, stop wearing 'normal' socks and instead wear trainer socks with ventilation panels throughout the whole year, including the winter months, and wear memory foam slippers. In regard to shoes, as my Grandma who was manager of a Saxone shoe shop years ago, used to say, "Your shoes should be designed to fit your feet and not your head", in other words, don't get shoes that look fashionable, but get ones that are practical for the care of your feet and good for your body. If the shoes you are looking at buying, are pointed at the toe, squash your feet because they are not wide enough, have a high heel that naturally shifts your pelvis forward, don't get them, as they will cause you pain. I get my shoes from Hotter, they are practical and roomy for your toes, and have very supportive soles and their aftercare service has been great so far. I am not saying Hotter shoes are right for you, as everybody's feet and experience is different and you need to find shoes that are right for you. I just thought you would like to know what works for me.

Because my tummy is also sensitive to pressure, I will often get the next size up in PJs and sometimes trousers too, to stop my clothes feeling like they are pressing on me and causing me pain. The objective is to be as pain free as possible, to feel good and be happy.

Because fibro can make you have a weak bladder and bowel, if this is an issue for you, its imperative to carry a spare set of underwear with you just in case you have an accident and you may want sanitary protection too. Some people take tablets for this and if they work and are not causing you any side effects and there is no better alternative, why not.

KEY POINTS TO REMEMBER

Your clothes can hurt you; make sure they are roomy enough to not be pressing on your pressure points. Get the next size up if you need to.

Wear trainer socks with ventilation panels throughout the whole year to stop your feet from swelling.

Wear memory foam slippers, no other type of slippers, to stop your feet from swelling.

Get shoes to fit your feet, not your head.

If you have a weak bladder or bowel, take spare underwear and/or sanitary protection with you wherever you go.

CHAPTER 16
WEATHER OR NOT HERE I COME

Some people with fibromyalgia often say the weather affects their degree of pain and the cold makes it worse. I function better in heat but that may be because I have always felt the cold. Having said that, I find the heat works best for soothing my pain and even throughout most of the summer months I will have up to 3 hot water bottles in bed each night; one for my feet and two each side of my hips. If my feet and hips get cold, then I can't sleep, or get proper rest. A heat pack works far better for reducing any swelling, and especially to my neck, than any ice pack. But I also need the window open at night to sleep better. I need my body temperature to be warm to function and do work, but I also need a good supply of oxygen in the form of fresh air, to help keep myself energised and awake, and also to help me to go to sleep, and I know that is a bit of a contradiction, but hey, being a superhero rockstar means you are not 'normal' in the sense of the word anyway, and to be honest, I would never want to be normal, living up to that fallacy is impossible, but making your dreams come true and living life your way, is not! So sometimes I have the heating on, and the windows open!

I don't fear rain anymore. I used to get chest infections every year and worried about the cold and rain, but like a superhero, if I get caught in the rain, I have no fear of getting wet, I think it's nature and it won't hurt me.

More effective than an umbrella against the wet weather, are waterproof trousers and a waterproof jacket. The ones I get are lightweight so they don't cause me pain, highly breathable, with taped seams. This makes them super easy to carry and by wearing them both together, over clothes, it's like being in a cocoon of warmth and prevents cold getting to my bottom half.

KEY POINTS TO REMEMBER

A heat pack works far better for reducing any swelling, especially to the neck, than any ice pack.

Heat is good for pain, but you also need oxygen in the form of a window being open, to stay energised, awake, and to sleep better.

Use waterproof trousers and a waterproof jacket that are lightweight so they don't cause you pain, but they keep you warm and dry.

CHAPTER 17
CAREER AND HOBBIES

Despite the fact that some days I woke up in a lot of pain and thought how am I going to get through the day; working a day job I enjoyed, was worth getting out of bed for every morning. In fact, I had less conscious pain going to work; than I did when I sat at home procrastinating over doing work, and the human body is extremely resilient, more than we give it credit for. So it could be just a short time later and I would be fine, either my pain would have died down, or more likely, I would be unconscious of my pain again. Yes, I admit I procrastinate, even when I do a lot more than the average person. When I worked in my day job, I was being distracted and I could get out of my head when talking to customers and staff. My focus and attention, was not on my body, but elsewhere, and therefore I became unconscious and unaware of my pain. And yes, I am still working on reducing the time I procrastinate and improving myself in that respect. A doctor once said to me, it may be more painful going to work because of your fibromyalgia, but it is also better for your mind that you do that. Although I am now redundant from that job I loved, I agree it is better than staying at home and not working at all. Also the socialising aspect of work is important to easing your pain; getting out and about, interacting, communicating, and connecting with others; is so healthy for you, much more than staying indoors and dwelling on your pain. Having said that, since being redundant for some time now, I prefer working from home, as it allows me to indulge in my passions that make me feel alive; it enables me to live my life more for me, on my own terms, which in turn gives me a greater sense of satisfaction and pleasure, to make me have that feel good factor and be in less pain. I aim to be able to work from home full-time in the future, so that should my fibromyalgia pain get worse and I end up needing care, I can pay for it at home and not have to go out to work. If you have not done so already, it is really important to start planning financially for your future right now. Work out how you can create an income online using your skills, abilities and knowledge, that you have already acquired, or go and make it your mission to acquire them.

Whether you work or not, you should ensure you have hobbies that take your mind off your pain; make you feel alive, and give you happiness and pleasure. Creative pursuits are great for this, as they allow you to get really engrossed in something that distracts your mind from your pain, whilst giving you a sense of achievement, and sometimes you can turn those pursuits into an income. If creative pursuits aren't your thing, find something that is. As mentioned in a previous chapter, get into personal and professional development. Start watching personal and professional development videos to grow yourself. If you feel like you are making progress in your life and not stagnating, it will give your life a greater sense of purpose and meaning, giving you that feel good factor to ease your pain and make you feel like life is very much amazing and worth living.

KEY POINTS TO REMEMBER

It may be more painful going to work because of your fibromyalgia, but it is better for your mind that you do that, rather than stagnating at home not doing any work at all.

The socialising aspect of work is important to easing your pain; getting out and about, interacting, communicating, and

connecting with others; is so healthy for you, much more than staying indoors and dwelling on your pain.

Start planning financially for your future right now. Work out how you can create an online income using your skills, abilities and knowledge, that you have already acquired, or go and make it your mission to acquire them.

Ensure you have hobbies that take your mind off your pain; make you feel alive, and give you happiness and pleasure.

Creative pursuits allow you to get really engrossed in something that distracts your mind from your pain, whilst giving you a sense of achievement, and sometimes you can turn those pursuits into an income.

If you feel like you are making progress in your life it will give you that feel good factor to ease your pain and make you feel like life is very much amazing and worth living.

CHAPTER 18
INTUITION AND YOUR MISSION

So something that isn't much talked about in relation to pain, is your core beliefs about who you are, what you are doing in this world, and what drives you in your life. Essentially your goals, ambitions and dreams – Your mission, that is your WHY and your purpose of what you are doing here in this world.

I have always known from a very young age, that I am different, and that I am born for a special purpose in life, it was the only thing that gave me hope and kept me going forward into the future whilst being depressed for years because I was bullied and in unhealthy relationships. I frequently hated my life, I felt upset; lonely, and misunderstood a lot of the time. So know now, you have a special purpose in life, everyone does whether they are consciously aware of it or not, and it is never too late to discover it and obtain it.

When you are older, you have the power of choice, the power to decide what is right and wrong for you and where you are headed in your life. You have the power to walk away from those situations that are no good for you; that are holding you back and creating bad energy for you in your life.

We don't always give our gut feeling the voice that it deserves. When we work against our gut feeling, we zap some of our energy, and a bit of our inner soul and being gets crushed in the process, which can result in anxiety in the body and pain. Of course, we have to assess if it really is a gut feeling, or if it is a fear we have and our brain is trying to trick us into not going near it because of the pain we may experience as a result of going through that fear. However, if you are in a job or situation that is no good for you, you will always have this sense that there is something more, that something is not quite right, and that you are not living up to your full potential. The solution is to find things to do, a job, hobbies, and situations to be in, that nourish your soul, that make you feel alive and that your life is worth living. That feel in tune with who you are and what you want to do in your life and that you feel rewarded for just by doing it, because it's who you are and you could not imagine yourself without it, it's central to your core being. When you are in tune with who you are and what you were born to be, you will have a greater sense of fulfilment, satisfaction, achievement, inner peace and happiness. Which in turn makes you feel good, gives you pleasure that you are loved by yourself and life, and gives you a deep sense of faith and comfort, that everything will work out well and that you are where you need to be right now in your life. When you feel this inner peace, your body is calmer, more relaxed and in less pain, thereby improving your overall health and wellbeing. So trust your own instincts, your judgement, and be confident in yourself, in your skills and your abilities. There lies within you, an incredible mind, which holds extreme power beyond your wildest beliefs, everyone has it; just most never access it, as they only use 10% of their brain. But you can learn to access it, through personal and professional development, which changed my life and made me see that I can learn whatever I put my mind to. It helped me to be in touch with my inner being. If your inner being is calling to you, then let it speak, it may just know what is best for you, better than you do. Sometimes you just have to take that leap of faith and go for something if it feels right and good for you, even if you are not sure how it will turn out, as life is way too short.

KEY POINTS TO REMEMBER

You have a special purpose in life and it is never too late to discover it and obtain it.

When you are older, you have the power of choice, the power to decide what is right and wrong for you and where you are headed in your life. You have the power to walk away from those situations that are no good for you; that are holding you back and creating bad energy for you in your life.

When we work against our gut feeling, we zap some of our energy, and a bit of our inner soul and being gets crushed in the process, which can result in anxiety in the body and pain.

If you are in a job or situation that is no good for you, you will always have this sense that there is something more, that something is not quite right and that you are not living up to your full potential.

When you are in tune with who you are and what you were born to be, you will have a greater sense of fulfilment, satisfaction, achievement, and inner peace and happiness, making you feel good, pleasure, loved by yourself and life, and having a deep sense of faith and comfort, that everything will work out well and that you are where you need to be right now in your life. When you feel this inner peace, your body is calmer, more relaxed and in less pain, thereby improving your overall health and wellbeing.

Trust your own instincts, your judgement, and be confident in yourself, in your skills and your abilities.

Sometimes you just have to take that leap of faith and go for something if it feels right and good for you, even if you are not sure how it will turn out.

CHAPTER 19
LOVE, RELATIONSHIPS, PHYSICAL
INTIMACY AND SEX

Something else I don't see spoken about in public, is how people who have fibromyalgia, cope with having physical intimacy with their partner. If your body is in pain, it is unlikely you are going to want to have sex, and in some cases, some people who have fibromyalgia can't have sexual intercourse at all because it hurts far too much and the anxiety of having to perform just creates more anguish and pain in their body, so this is a time when sex could actually be very bad for your health and should be avoided. Some people choose to refrain from having intercourse and do other things such as oral sex or masturbate their partner. Some become disinterested in it, and some people put up with the pain through intercourse for the sake of their partner. Let's discuss in greater detail, your options to reduce your pain and discomfort, and what to do if it hurts too much to have sex at all.

If you are a woman there are steps you can take to reduce the pain such as being wet before you have intercourse through masturbation. You could either masturbate yourself if you find that more comfortable, as you know your pain points better than anyone else, or what you may find far more satisfying and sexually pleasing to both you and your partner, is to show and explain to them, EXACTLY what turns you on, how and where you like to be touched, licked, kissed and sucked, to make you extremely wet and in the least pain possible. So they masturbate you and do as much foreplay as possible to get you wet. The wetter the better, for decreasing the amount of pain you will be in during intercourse. If something hard (his penis), is rubbing against something dry – your vagina if you are not wet, that is going to cause friction and hurt you. If something hard, is going into something wet, soft and squishy, it's going to fit in with far more ease and less pain. That's why making love in a Jacuzzi, can feel far more pleasurable and give you far less pain, or a swimming pool, because the water really helps slipping in with ease and the water is soothing. It can also be both a thrilling and exciting experience to make love in a different environment than a bed. Give your partner the challenge of trying to make you as wet, comfortable, and in as least pain as possible for intercourse, or you really can't have it! This is an opportunity for your partner to explore your body, but with your own guidance, and really step up to the plate to make you have the most physical pleasure, remember the antidote to feeling pain, is to feel pleasure. You need to put your own pleasure needs first where your fibro and sexual intercourse is concerned, because if all you feel is pain and you become fearful of intercourse because of that, you are not going to want to have it at all. The ONLY way you are going to even want sexual intercourse, is if your partner makes it a good experience for you. Remember the antidote to feeling bad, is to feel good.

Foreplay is essential to making you wet, but it doesn't have to lead to sexual intercourse; you could finish off by masturbating him, or not. If you are too tired and in pain, let him do that for himself. Remember, you ALWAYS have the right to say NO or STOP to doing any sexual acts and intercourse, at any time, even if your partner is about to cum. I have done this in the past and didn't feel guilty at all. This was before my fibromyalgia diagnosis, when sex still hurt probably more often than not. My partner at that time, was good at making me in the least amount of pain possible, because he was great at all the foreplay stuff, and he experimented with different positions of sexual intercourse, which I highly rec-ommend you do. Experiment with different sexual positions to find which ones are the more comfortable for you. Get a book about different sex positions if it will help you, or Google 'different sex positions'. I found being on the bed, but turning on my side, sometimes really helped lessen the pain, or going on top of a guy (if you are into guys), and just riding on the tip of his penis rather than going all in, was much better, as it was less painful because I could control the amount of penetration and the depth of it. If you are in a relationship and developed fibro since you got together, it is essential you communicate with your partner even more than before your diagnosis, to see how each other's needs can be met, and explore ways around it. You might find you need to adapt var-ious sex positions by using more cushions to support you. Even without sex, fibromyalgia can make your body shake and this can be visible or feel like internal shaking which can't be seen, so this needs to be explained to your partner and needs understanding from them.

If you are not keen on the idea of masturbation to get wet, or you want an alternative, you could try lube for lubrication of your vagina or his penis, before you have sexual intercourse. But if you are sensitive to any of the ingredients in it, or become allergic or sensitive to any of them, which may well happen with fibro as you know it can make your body and skin sensitive to many things, then it will cause you more discomfort. If you are using condoms for birth control, or to prevent STIs and STDs, you can buy latex free condoms, if you are allergic to latex.

Mutual masturbation can be a great alternative to penetrative sex, but this can make your hands and wrists ache, so it's best to find a comfortable position that works for you and gives you the least amount of pain and discomfort. If you are in too much pain to have sex and you also don't want to be on the receiving end of mastur-bation, tell your partner this, be direct with them. You may still want to masturbate your partner, if you feel up to it. You could give them a massage, or still lick, kiss and suck, your partner's ero-genous zones; you could fondle their genitals, or if they are female, suck their breasts; explore their body and still have fun. Just make it clear what is and isn't off limits.

To give and receive oral sex is another alternative to penetrative sex. However, be aware that oral sex can give you thrush, which is an infection that can be painful. Oh and it's okay to spit his semen out if you can't swallow it, or take your mouth away just before he is about to explode his load. Don't feel bad about this. The more you have fun having sex and doing sexual acts, the more you be your authentic self and do what feels right to you and is good for you, the less pain and discomfort you will be in and that will be great for both of you. As a woman it is okay to assert yourself and tell your partner what you want. It is okay for you to be the more dominant one in the sex positions if it helps you to be in less pain or you just enjoy it more that way. If you find it too strenuous to be the one in the more dominant position, then get your partner to do more of the work. They need to work hard to make sex and sex acts comfortable for you, if they can't do that, then they won't get the sexual reward they want, so it's in their interests to make it work.

Some women have an over-sensitive clitoris and find direct clitoral pressure too intense for prolonged stimulation, so too much mas-turbation, or done in the wrong way for your body, can feel very bad to you, and you won't be able to do much of it and it could make your vagina too sensitive for sexual intercourse. Besides the clitoris, there are other parts of the vagina that can give you physi-cal pleasure and make you wet and cum. There is something known as the G Spot and O Spot, Google 'G Spot and O Spot' to find out more about these, and explore your body to find out what works for you. No two bodies or relationships are the same and you shouldn't be comparing yours to other people.

Talk to your partner and explain what feels good and right for you. Sex and physical intimacy needs and preferences, should be discussed between you and your partner, in a non-threatening, relaxed, and approachable manner. Your partner should be someone who loves and cares deeply for you and about your health and wellbeing. They should be someone who respects you and your boundaries and who wants to please you, satisfy you, make you feel safe, comfortable and happy, whilst also loving themselves and caring about their own health and wellbeing. They should be your best friend and you should be able to talk to them with ease, and without fear. They should be sensitive to your needs and sympathetic and compassionate towards your feelings and emotions. They should be caring and kind and put your emotional wellbeing and physical needs above their own sexual desires. Your partner should make your comfort a priority and your feelings should be of the utmost importance to them. When you love someone, you hold their heart in your hand, so it's important that your partner wants to protect it and keep it safe.

Intimacy is not just about sex and sexual acts, it's about a deep emotional connection and bond with each other, feeling safe in each other's company and that you can talk about anything and everything with your partner. It should be about sharing secrets with each other, sharing your hopes, dreams and fears. You should be growing together and supporting growth in each other as individuals. You should both be willing to improve your own self, in order to make the relationship the best it can be. Working on a creative project together, saving up for a dream trip together, talking about the world, planet and universe, with nothing off limits, and building a business together, are all forms of intimacy, because it takes a great deal of trust and vulnerability to share those things with each other, not just your body, but your mind, emotions, deepest desires and your soul.

If you don't have an understanding partner, and especially where sex and physical intimacy is concerned, the whole experience is going to be more traumatic than pleasurable, and this type of situation has to change, or you won't be having any sex without it hurting you – which in turn will make your fibromyalgia pain so much worse. Whether you are married, in a relationship, or dating, and having sex or doing sexual acts, when you don't enjoy it and don't want to do it because it doesn't feel good to you, and especially being pressured into thinking it's your fault and you are being selfish, it's not right and it is abuse. If you are constantly being put down and belittled because of your disability, it becomes emotionally abusive, which is why you will be forever getting severe fibro flare ups, swelling and pain. If you have tried your best to communicate with your partner, to work around those difficulties and they are not listening and making you feel bad and the relationship is becoming painful for you to be in, you need to leave it. Yes, I said leave. There is no point in two people continuing to be together if they are making each other miserable and that misery will manifest itself in acute debilitating body pain, lethargy, and illness. You will find you are no longer living life but just surviving within it, and that may make you feel like you won't be able to get anyone else for a relationship, but that simply isn't true, many people have disabilities but are still in relationships. It's the situation you are in, which is making you so very ill and it's better to be single, than be in a perpetual state of pain from the anxiety, emotional upset, and depression of such a situation. So yes, I am saying leave, separate, and get divorced if you need to. Think you did the best you could, but you have the right to change your mind and walk away. Life is too short, and while you are with the wrong person, the right person will not come along, and your fibromyalgia pain will not decrease, but do the opposite. Or you become so numb in the relationship, that you will no longer recognise yourself, believe me, I have been there, and those years I cannot get back, but the freedom I have now was well worth leaving those relationships behind. Those traumatic relationships contributed to me getting fibromyalgia, especially the last one for 8.5 years, I think that was what finally pushed me into a state of having it. I have it for life, those guys don't, they get to walk away free in that respect. I take responsibility that I chose to be with them and I did not walk away sooner. Yes I felt financially reliant on them, but even when I walked away the first time from that last one after 1.5 years, after him stalking me, I still got back with him 6 months later for another 7 years, making a total of 8.5 years. I lacked self-love back then and felt like he had a magnetic hold over me, I also lacked fibromyalgia. As I mentioned before, fibromyalgia has become my weapon and superpower in the fight against ever being with such guys ever again. One of the last times he ever accidentally on purpose turned up outside my home – which is the opposite side of the city to where he lives, I had just been diagnosed with fibromyalgia, and he proceeded to tell me about how he was going into the hospital to finally have the lump near his nipple removed, which I had been telling him he should go and see a doctor about for the majority of two years when I was with him. As soon as I said I have fibromyalgia, a disability for life, it was one of the things that completely turned him off from getting back into a relationship with me or pursuing me ever again; which I was glad about, as I never wanted to get back with him and I didn't want him to pursue me. When I was with him, any time I was feeling ill, which I felt quite a lot whilst being in a toxic relationship with him, he always had to have an illness worse that mine, and fibromyalgia, as a disability for life, he could not compete with. That was the way he would have seen it. He was abusive in every way but sexually. So fibromyalgia is truly life saving for me, as I won't get and stay in a relationship like that ever again, and have so much more self-love and enjoy the freedom of being single. It may be that your partner is not abusive, but you just cannot make it work any longer, and you are constantly upset and in pain over the situation, if that is the case, it's sad, but the relationship can't go on forever like it, your fibromyalgia will be consistently flaring up, because that emotional pain will definitely manifest itself in your body as pain and neither of you will end up happy, and you are both wasting your life so need to split up.

If you have fibromyalgia, are currently single, and experience acute pain that prevents you from ever having sex and you feel you will never get a partner who can love you without sex, you may be interested to know that there is a sexual orientation called asexuality, that is the lack of sexual attraction, you can check out this site that is the biggest online community for asexuals, www.asexuality.org, to find out more, and take a look at my own site www.asexualise.com and my channel where I educate people about asexuality www.youtube.com/asexualisemyasexuallife. Essentially, asexuals do not get the need, urge, or want, for partnered sexual intercourse, so they don't have to have sex, to have a long lasting, loving, healthy, happy relationship. Some romantic asexuals like me, still want romance, kissing and cuddling, without the sex. I am fortunate in that I discovered I am a heteroromantic asexual (romantically attracted to the opposite sex – guys, but not sexually), before my pain got so bad that I can no longer have sexual intercourse as it would likely be too painful for me, because that is one of the worst affected pain areas of my body. Well that is what the nurse and me agreed on, that it would be too painful for me to have sexual intercourse these days. Although I always think where there's a will, there's a way, and maybe if I desperately wanted sex I could find a way, such as being very wet and riding on top of a guy 'occasionally', that way I could control the depth of penetration, that wouldn't usually be frequently enough to satisfy most heterosexual guys, and the point is, as an asexual that does not experience sexual attraction and does not desire sex – I had sex in the past because that is what I thought I was meant to do as part of a 'normal' relationship, there is no will to have it in the first place, and I don't want to put my body through that again. When I had sex in the past, before I realised I am asexual and before my fibromyalgia diagnosis, because my ex was good at foreplay and being wet really helped to lessen the pain, it was not too bad, although from an asexual point of view, I would rather have not had sex as I don't associate sex with love or ever have a need for it in my life. I want to reiterate, don't ever have sex if it hurts and you don't want to do it. Married or not, in a relationship or not, if a person is having sex when they don't want to, it's wrong. You need to be as pain free and happy as possible and if your partner can't understand that and they would rather you put up with the pain for their own sexual desires, and discussing things with them is not working, it's time to move on from that relationship, otherwise it will be the cause of your pain, because you will feel anxious whenever they are being very affectionate with you, that it will lead to another painful sex session and your body just can't take that any more. I refuse to date heterosexuals anymore, because I am asexual and heterosexuals usually always need sex at some point in their life. So unless I met a guy that could genuinely be 100% sex free and happy and never cheat, I will only date asexual guys now. I even wrote a book about asexuality that is available on Amazon in digital format and paperback, <u>Asexual Perspectives 47 Asexual Stories, Love Life and Sex, ACElebration of Diversity</u>. I interviewed 46 asexuals around the globe for this book and I also share my own personal story in the book too. So if you are a sexual person, such as a heterosexual, rather than an asexual person, and you can't have sex because of your fibromyalgia, know that there are people out there who will love you for who you are and not leave you for not being able to have sex. Just be honest with them as to your reason for wanting a relationship without sex and don't pretend to be asexual if you are not, let them know it is your fibromyalgia preventing you from having sex as the thinking about sex and attitude towards it can be very different. You may want it in theory, just not be able to have it in practice, whereas we don't usually think about it or desire it in the first place.

KEY POINTS TO REMEMBER

If your body is in pain, it is unlikely you are going to want to have sex, and in some cases, some people who have fibromyalgia can't have sexual intercourse at all because it hurts far too much and the anxiety of having to perform, just creates more anguish and pain in their body.

Some people put up with the pain through intercourse for the sake of their partner, while others choose to refrain from having intercourse and do other things such as oral sex or masturbate their partner.

If you are a woman with fibromyalgia and you want to have sexual intercourse, making sure you are very wet before you have it, can make the experience a lot less painful for you. So either masturbate yourself, or get your partner to do that for you, and do lots of other foreplay to get you wet and make the whole experience as fun, pleasurable, and sexually satisfying as possible. Experiment with different positions to find out

what makes you have the least amount of pain and discomfort as possible, and adapt those if you need to. Consider going on top of the guy, so you can control the depth of penetration.

If sexual intercourse is too painful and not an option, consider giving and receiving oral sex and mutual masturbation, or you could masturbate your partner and give them oral sex, without it being reciprocated.

You should never have sex if you don't want to.

Don't stay in a relationship that is causing you more pain.

If you have fibromyalgia, are currently single, and you feel you will never get a partner who can love you without sex, there is a sexual orientation called asexuality, that is the lack of sexual attraction, and asexuals can have loving, healthy, happy relationships, without sex ever. Check out my blog for asexuals at www.asexualise.com and the biggest online community for asexuals at www.asexuality.org. For more information about asexuality and to gain a deeper understanding about it, watch and subscribe to my channel about asexuality here www.youtube.com/asexualisemyasexuallife and buy a copy of Asexual Perspectives 47 Asexual Stories, Love Life and Sex, ACElebration of Diversity on Amazon or www.sellfy.com/quirkybooks.net You can also request the printed edition of this book from all good book shops around the globe, as it's published under my own imprint of Quirky Books so they can order it in for you.

If you approach an asexual for a relationship, be honest that you are not asexual but it is your fibromyalgia that prevents you from having sex!

CHAPTER 20
LIVE LIKE A TEENAGER

Remember when you were a teenager and you had no fear; you would try new things and enjoy life to the max, because why not? Remember you would most likely have the most awesome bedroom filled with the most amazing toys, sparkly things, bright lights and coloured boxes, pretty things, and bizarre things? It would be filled up with a collection of stuff that is most precious to you and that you enjoyed using or playing with. Do you remember that? Your wallpaper may have looked like something cute and cuddly, or alien, or adventure like, and you would find your room was packed to the brim of both stuff you were using and stuff you had no real interest in, but it looked cool at the time. Essentially, it was a young and vibrant place, full of fantasy, energy, imagination, and promise of dreams coming true. It was a space that you could feel was your own, and it had character because you stamped your character all over it. Contrast that with your 'adult' bedroom, which may be bland, consisting of a couple of blocks of colour, a few books and keepsakes, but in general it is clean, tidy, and more formal. It looks like everything is in its place and minimalistic. But what is missing is that energy, that vibrancy, that cute and cuddliness; that magic where dreams are made and they come true. Essentially your childhood essence has been depleted and along with it, your childhood hopes, dreams, vitality, vibrancy, and no fear attitude; that you can tackle anything in life that comes your way. You have lost that feeling of thriving and of being alive in the moment, with the magic of life, in the now.

You need to take back that sense of wonder and amazement, that feeling of dreams coming true, and stop living as an 'adult', in an unstimulated and uninspired environment and live your life for you. This is key to reducing your fibro pain. I live like a 15-year-old teenager in my home environment and love it. I also purposefully have a 21-year-old mindset, (I refer to this as my 21st mindset), which improves my quality of life incredibly and I will be telling you more about that later in this book. I don't care what people think, because it keeps me young and feeling energetic, vibrant, happy, and full of life, and reminds me that anything is possible; life is magical and never give up! It is this attitude and mindset that enables me to do far more than many others with fibro, it's great, and I get to experience the magic and wonder of life and of dreams coming true, every single day of my life. I wake up to the sound of my Iron Man alarm clock going off, and me having to press his head to snooze the light. I go to sleep with my Winnie the Pooh and Piglet bedside lamp on. I get to experience the cute and colourful cuddly toys that are spread around my bedroom and sleep with me on the other side of my double bed. I get to see a sparkly heart and bauble, a fibre optic lamp and brightly coloured boxes. I love life and it loves me back. I have kids books and watch kids movies. I am a kid and I nourish my inner child. What are you doing to nourish your inner child?

Environment is not just about one room in your home, such as your bedroom, it is about ensuring each room in your home is giving you as much energy and happiness as it possibly can. It is about having your favourite things around you, your favourite colours, furniture and fabrics. It's about what makes you feel good. That may be playing your favourite music; having your favourite pictures on the wall and ornaments on shelves in your room; pets; plants; hobby stuff, or anything that makes you smile.

The mind is more powerful than the body, so long as you keep exercising that; it is the most important thing and environment overall. A dead mind, is like a dead soul, so whatever mobility issues you may have, remember to keep your brain active as much as possible on a consistent daily basis. When my Grandma was in a nursing home, although I was not happy with the condition she was being kept in some of the time, and I attended meetings expressing my concerns, what was even worse, was the fact they stopped her from walking by telling her she needed to use a wheelchair all the time even after her leg had healed from her fall, so she was restricted by what they allowed her to do and they stopped doing activities with her, which made her mind go dead. My Grandma was diagnosed with an overactive brain when young; she used to get up in the early hours and write sums on the wall. Before her fall, when she was in her own home, she used to walk around, make herself do stuff and use wordsearches to keep her brain active. She would recite past events and keep her brain going. When she first went into the nursing home they had activities to do, but sadly these got less and less, until one Easter they advertised an event that looked great to visitors of the residents, but never happened because I was there. So although she got a 'cold' and had throat problems, I believe this was the real cause of her dying at 96, because her active brain was essential to the life of my Grandma's being; it was core to who she was. I am thankful and grateful to have had her that long and been with her at the end. But I will always learn my greatest lessons from her, "There is no such word as can't," and "If you don't use it, you lose it", and you should apply those to your own life in managing your fibro.

Now I am free of bad relationships and live life how I want to live – like a young teenager, life is super awesome. I look younger, feel younger, and am truly living my life and feel alive and invigorated. I have so much more energy, more ambition than ever before, and

I am in touch with my soul and life missions and making them happen. I couldn't be happier in that respect.

A lot of people with fibro find it hard to sleep and this can cause negativity and depression. In the next chapter I am going to show you how to handle your sleep problem like a superhero rockstar so you can start to feel great again.

KEY POINTS TO REMEMBER

Adopt a teenager lifestyle and don't care what people think. Unleash your inner child and get back to having dreams and feeling alive again, choose to have a home environment that is full of life, energy, and things that give you pleasure and make you feel good.

A dead mind equates to a dead soul, so keep your mind active at all times.

Do things in spite of your pain. Remember my Grandma's golden rules, "There is no such word as can't", and "If you don't use it you lose it".

PART 5
HOW TO MANAGE YOUR SLEEP LIKE A SUPERHERO ROCKSTAR!

CHAPTER 21
HOW TO DO THE WRONG THING
TO GET THE RIGHT RESULT

Rockstars live life to the max, they do what they love and they live their life their way. They are not dictated to by society or social norms or conventions, and they don't care what people think.

It is common for people who have fibromyalgia to have insomnia and sleep problems, and it is often hard to get that deep sleep we need to feel refreshed, awake and alive!

It is well known by society that medical professionals recommend 8 hours of sleep a day and this is expected to be carried out before midnight, through until the next morning. You are expected to either lie there until you drop off to sleep, or to find things to make you feel calmer and relaxed to send you off to sleep. Relaxation music; meditation; breathing techniques; a warm milky drink before bed (try herbal tea if you are lactose or dairy free); reading a book, switching the computer screen or TV off an hour before bed, and keeping a diary of your thoughts and feelings, can help, but the problem is, they don't work for everyone, or not necessarily in the same way, and the bigger problem is what we are expected to do, and how and when we are expected to do it. Remember when I said at the beginning of this book that I manage fibromyalgia very unconventionally, I have a ton of energy, can go out to theme parks, zoos, aquariums, clubbing, and live life to the max! This is because I don't do what I am told to do, I do what works for me. I don't listen to society's norms, when they don't work for me. You have to embrace your quirky and live for you.

As a rule, when I was working in a day job, I didn't go to bed early, usually after 2.30am, sometimes 3.30am. I am a creative night owl who comes alive at night and I have far more energy and focus at night than in the day, and I am usually far more productive at that time. Which means that when I went to my day job and had to get up at 7.30am, sometimes I only had 3-4 hours sleep a night. So after 4 nights of this pattern, I would have a lie in on my day off by sleeping longer during the morning and afternoon, and if I needed to go to bed very early one night I did, but in doing that, I would usually be more lethargic and lacking energy the next day.

Before I was made redundant, one night I went to bed really early and had over 11 hours sleep to make up for the lack of sleep in recent days. But when I got up at the time I would usually get up for my day job, by 3pm I had pounding ear pain that went down the side of my face. I took Ibuprofen that did nothing for the pain, and I had to live with it for hours whilst doing a big food shop. I can also get ear pain from a lack of sleep but still have a lot of energy, whereas with this amount of sleep, I felt like I had a lack of energy and I felt older. I went to bed and the next morning my head was worse than before and thumping and I had to cancel an appointment. I could only put this down to having too much sleep at the wrong time for me. I changed back to sleeping later in the early hours and had far more energy and vibrancy and was living life to the max again. I am backwards in this respect, but this is me; it's who I am. Before I was made redundant, I worked out the best time for me to go to sleep in the morning is 4am and wake up at midday, that still gives me 8 hours of sleep, but not just any sleep, that deep, quality sleep, that most fibro sufferers lack (although sometimes I don't need that much sleep because I naturally wake up having far less), which was great when I was not working in my day job, but meant on a work day I wouldn't get much sleep before it, if I didn't go to sleep until after 3am. If society, doctors, and the world we live in, stopped trying to tell people there is something wrong with them, that they have a disorder if they don't fit into a specific box, and instead say it's okay to work with the natural rhythm of your body, to work with your own gut feelings and intuition, and to trust your own instincts more, and value your own worth for being an individual, I believe there would be far less people in distressed emotional states, far less people labelled with mental health disorders, and more people being happy with who they are and satisfied with their life. We have to ask ourselves, are these people who are determining if we have a disorder and constantly saying there is something wrong with us if we don't do this or that, a product of conditioning? Personally, I could not think of anything worse than going to bed regularly at 10.30pm, that makes me feel like an old woman and like I am not experiencing life. Remember, the goal is to decrease your pain and to have more energy, so you need to do what is right for you and your body and if that means doing the wrong thing, to get the right result, such as sleeping in the day, and being awake throughout the night so you can get a better quality of sleep, then so be it!

SUPERHERO MINDSET

Overall, I have a superhero mindset where sleep is concerned, I don't believe I need tons of it; I believe quality of sleep is far more important. I would rather get 4-6 hours of deep sleep, than lie awake for an hour trying to go to sleep. Why are people wasting their life away doing this? What is the point of lying in bed doing nothing? How is that going to make you feel good, happy, and give you pleasure? Always remember that antidote quote. If what you are doing is not giving you any of those 6 antidotes, making you feel good; happy; pleasure; loved; safe; and having faith, stop doing it! Live your life how you are meant to, not how anyone else thinks you should live it. There is a deep-rooted fear that if we don't get enough sleep, it is so bad for our health and this or that may happen as a result. Do superheroes need 8 hours sleep everyday? No, they sleep when they are able to and want to, but use their inner powers to live with energy and vitality. They develop a way of living at night, when activity is usually at its highest. There are times when I have to force myself to stay up and work, and I often use club, dance, and techno music to energise myself to do this, as well as using those to energise myself in the day when at home. But sometimes, that very same music, I can also use to send me off to sleep, yes, you did hear right, I can use dance music to make me fall peacefully off to sleep. Admittedly, there are some times I am so tired from a lack of sleep, that I can't keep my eyes open and I start to fall asleep at my desk and I have to go immediately to sleep, but this is great because I am so 'knocked out with tiredness' I get a much deeper and better quality of sleep, and this makes me feel amazing if I don't get too much sleep.

As for lying in bed trying to get to sleep when you can't, this is a huge NO, NO, NO, for a fibro sufferer, because you will suffer, so if you find yourself doing this – stop it now. Yet this is what we are told to do, lie down until you fall asleep, get some rest and get plenty of sleep. Staying in bed draws attention to my pain, so I do the opposite of that and feel alive, energetic, vibrant, good and happy. When you lie there, you can feel your pain because you become more consciously aware of it, and that is absolutely no good for your mind, it will hurt you if you do this and you will feel your pain. Get up, get moving, and do some stuff. Watch a movie, go PM a friend on Facebook, go get out of your head, stay awake until you 'feel' tired and 'need' to sleep, then go to sleep. Do the opposite of what you have been taught to do, don't go to bed to sleep, go to bed when you actually feel tired and need to sleep; not when it is expected, but when it feels right for you. This is how you become far more productive each day. People may make you feel bad for not going to sleep at a 'reasonable hour', but they are the ones missing out on life, not you, while they are forcing themselves to go to sleep, you are living your natural sleep pattern, you are experiencing life, whereas they are going through the motions because that is what they have been conditioned to do. Don't do what the majority do, do what's right and feels good for you, and don't care what people think, you are your own person and you have more inner power and strength within you than you realise. If you have sleep problems and find it hard to get to sleep, experiment with times of going to sleep, try going to sleep later or at some hour that most people would find strange. Sleep in the day and get up at night if that works well for you. Or try falling asleep on top of your bed, when your mind does not feel pressurised to go to bed and sleep when it's expected to, this works well for me, as does keeping a bedside light on because I don't like the dark and sometimes listening to some meditations on YouTube.

I personally get a buzz out of going to bed in the early hours and having less sleep than most, I sleep when I want and get up with a spring in my step. In my mind I have always disliked sleep and thought it is a pointless waste of time and life, and if I can spend more hours awake and be more productive and get stuff done, I feel happy and good about that and have less pain because of that mindset. I know I have to get some sleep though, as it is good for the body to have some rest for it's proper functioning, I just prefer it not to be before midnight and at a time that feels good to me, then if I get 8 hours or more of sleep, I know it's deep quality sleep and I will wake up feeling refreshed and re-energised for the day ahead.

Since being made redundant I have predominantly been going to sleep between 2.30am and 4am, sometimes I work through the night until 7.30am and then go to sleep. Many times I just get up when I wake up naturally and don't set my alarm unless I need to get up or go out for a very specific reason. Just listen to your own body and do what works for you and know that it's okay to defy conventions. Know it's okay if you sleep longer sometimes as your body needs a rest; so long as you wake up refreshed, revitalised and energised, and don't stay there lying in bed in pain and wide awake as that will zap your energy. Go to bed when you literally feel like dropping to sleep, and know it's okay to have fewer hours of sleep.

If you are currently sharing a bed with someone and can't sleep, it's likely because they are near your pressure points and you need a bigger bed or a separate bed. We are going to discuss what makes a good bed for your fibro condition in the next chapter, but right now I feel I need to tell you about some of the side effects and problems with having little sleep, so here goes:

- You need to eat more for sustained energy throughout the day and night, and this can make you put on weight which is hard to get off again.

- You can develop digestive problems because you are eating late at night to stay awake, energised and focused.

- You can get chest pains, which may make you feel like you are going to have a heart attack, or there is something seriously wrong with you – but you just need to get more sleep.

- Your body feels like it hasn't rested and can feel achier.

- You can feel tired at the most inappropriate times.

- You may get headaches and feel dizzy.

- You have to keep yourself constantly energised through music, movement, food and water.

- It can be hard to concentrate and focus on certain tasks that require more than average brainpower, such as problem solving, so you may need to leave these tasks for when you feel more awake and that could be inconvenient if the task is urgent or critical – you will have to access your super survival state just to complete it and give sufficient energy to it to get it done to the best of your ability in that state, and this requires you to expel less energy and conserve energy on other tasks. So you cut down talking to people, leave housework and moving around doing other stuff, and literally just be super attention giving to the task at hand and pretend you have curtains around you, so that almost everything else is blocked out.

- You may get more emotional or become more sensitive to things people say.

- You may close yourself off to loved ones and friends, because you don't feel like talking as much and/or to conserve your energy for important tasks, and this could be damaging to your relationship with them. So it's essential you keep communicating with them and let them know when you need to focus more on other stuff, or need down time, or space to yourself. Ensure you factor some time in to spend with them as and when you can, put it on your calendar and in your diary, so they know they have your ultimate time and attention for that certain time and stick to it.

You may have more to add to this list, as it is by no means exhaustive, so you need to work out whether having less sleep than most, is beneficial to you. If I am at home and my legs feel more jelly like and I start to feel they need an elevated rest and I need some sleep, eventually, after I have finished what I am doing, or made enough progress with it, I will go and get some. If I have less sleep, but feel more energetic, happier, more alive, and in less conscious pain, the pros outweigh the cons for me, but everyone is different. Although you may find, that like me, if sometimes you go to sleep at a much later hour, such as 4am, and wake up at midday, that you will get more sleep and deeper sleep and still get the recommended 8 hours of sleep. So consider not just the length of time you sleep for, but the quality of that sleep and how it eases your pain or makes it worse, then make your decision as to how much sleep you personally need, based on those results.

KEY POINTS TO REMEMBER

Don't go to bed to sleep, go to bed when you actually feel tired and need to sleep.

Don't stay in bed trying to get to sleep, get up and get moving, and do some stuff until you need to sleep.

Experiment with the time you go to sleep, even if it's 4am in the morning.

Don't be fearful of having less than 8 hours sleep. It is better to have 4-6 hours of quality, deep sleep, than to try going to bed at an expected 'reasonable hour', and not being able to sleep for an hour and being consciously aware of your pain.

Don't do what society wants you to do with your sleep, do what's right for you.

CHAPTER 22
NIGHT, NIGHT, DON'T
SLEEP TIGHT!

Because fibro makes you sensitive to pressure points it's important to choose your mattress and bed wisely. Luckily for you I was the manager of a bed company for 3 years, and I worked next to a bed department in my last job for 5 years, so I have years of experience giving advice to people about beds and mattresses. So let's get one thing cleared up, it used to be said that having an orthopaedic firm mattress was good for a bad back; this is no longer the case. From my vast experience, getting the best mattress and bed for you is dependent on body weight and height. So in general, someone who is shorter and slimmer, needs something softer, than someone who is taller or heavier in weight, or who has a bigger body mass. The mattress should come up into the arch of your back to support you. If you get the wrong mattress, for example, you are short and slim and get a firm mattress, you will lie on it like a board and it will not support you, so you will get backache. If you are 20 stone and have a soft mattress, you will dip down in it and it won't be coming up into your arch to support you, do you see how this works? So you need to ensure you get the right tension for you. If you have a partner who you sleep in the same bed with and they are considerably different in body weight or height to you, you will be pleased to know that you can get some split tension beds, so this means that some beds will have a mattress that could be firm on one side and soft or medium on the other, just be mindful of this when you need to turn it to keep the fillings evened out to stop it getting lumpy and make it last longer, because you may find you have to swap sides if you rotate it. Most people find that a medium tension works best, but if you have fibromyalgia that makes you super sensitive to pressure, and you are not small or thin, but not huge either, you may need to add a mattress topper for an extra layer of comfort to a medium tension mattress, as the soft tension may be too soft for you and not come up into the arch of your back to support you, but it may be too firm for your pressure points. It is for this reason that memory foam mattresses are often recommended for fibro sufferers, as they are meant to relieve pressure because they have no springs, or fillings, and no tufts to hold fillings in place. Although you can get a mattress that has springs, (pocket sprung are considered the best) and a layer of memory foam on top, which would always be my preference if I was to have any sort of memory foam bed, because pure memory foam beds are too firm for me and I could not get on with just a memory foam pillow. I have an expensive handmade pocket sprung bed that has a lot of sumptuous fillings with no foam. A pocket sprung bed will always be a more supportive bed for you than a traditional open coil bed. With traditional open coil mattresses, all the springs are linked together, so if one spring goes down, so will the rest, meaning they do not come up into the arch of your back to support you and correctly align your spine like a pocket sprung mattress does, and if you are in bed with a partner, you will feel them moving around. With a pocket sprung bed, the springs are in their own individual pockets of material and move independently of each other, that means they are free to come up into the arch of your back to support you and you should not feel your partner moving around much. My bed is medium in tension but was the softest medium available at the time, it is getting older now and I began to feel the tufts in 2017. I also noticed I had more pressure points that were causing my back to hurt more, so my mum bought me a topper for it. I tried a memory foam one at first, but as it was inexpensive, the polyurethane fire retardancy stank my flat out and there was no way I could live like that, so I took it back. It did not feel right to me either. I now have a thick polyester one and it has made a huge difference to my quality of sleep, it is softer for me, and now I have less pain. I would always recommend getting the right mattress in the first place, so you don't need a topper, but with fibromyalgia, your tension and comfort needs may differ so you may find you need to add a topper as an extra comfort layer to relieve your pressure points. Essentially, you want your bed/mattress to be soft enough to relieve the pressure of your body pressure points, but supportive enough in tension to correctly align your spine and not cause you back or neck pain.

Remember to get a waterproof mattress protector to put over your mattress and topper, to keep them as clean and hygienic as possible. Also to keep them dry if you spill any liquids or have any accidents if you suffer from incontinence, which may be because of a weak bladder or bowel because of your fibromyalgia.

Never sit on the edge of your bed to tie your shoelaces or just because you feel like it, as this can damage your mattress and decrease its lifespan. If it gets damaged, it won't be supportive for you and therefore it will increase the pain you already have from your fibro. If you are going for a sprung mattress, go for one that is not only pocket sprung, but also one that is hand side stitched to give you total edge-to-edge support. This will mean you can lie (not sit), right on the edge of your bed and still have the springs support you underneath to keep your spine correctly aligned, as opposed to a machine side-stitched mattress, where the springs will splay out at the sides as there is nothing to hold them in place. Sometimes you may have to wait for 4-8 weeks for a handmade pocket sprung bed with hand side-stitching to be made, my bed took 6 weeks to make, but it was well worth the wait!

An alternative to a spring or memory foam mattress is a latex mattress. Unlike memory foam that takes some time to go back into shape, a latex mattress springs back into shape instantly. With memory foam, it is recommended you use a very low tog duvet, even in winter, or you can feel too hot in it. Natural latex is made from a natural rubber tree plant and dust mites can't usually live in latex, so it is better for allergy sufferers and you don't need to use a low tog duvet with it all the time either. Memory foam is also inhospitable to dust mites. So either of these will also make healthier and more supportive pillows than down or polyester fibre, which the dust mites love to live in. I have a <u>Dunlopillo Serenity latex pillow</u> and it provides amazing support for my neck and I only need one pillow. I tried a memory foam pillow with a roll under the neck on the advice of a physiotherapist, but it actually hurt my neck and I could not sleep with it, so I sold it.

Through my experience of managing a bed company for 3 years and getting involved in the bed department that was adjacent to my fitted bedroom department in my day job, I would avoid buying any pillow top mattress. Pillow top mattresses are usually single-sided mattresses, which have an extra comfort layer of fillings on top of the mattress and it looks like a topper, but is an integral part of the mattress and non-removable. This extra comfort layer may seem like a dream to a fibro sufferer, but it can become a nightmare, because these fillings, unlike latex or memory foam that spring back into shape, bed down with time, which can be within a matter of months, as the fillings naturally settle. This is called natural settlement, and is not a fault, but it can feel like one, because it often causes impressions of your body to be left in the mattress, that look like dips, and can feel like lumps or ridges, and be very uncomfortable. As it is a single-sided mattress, you can only rotate it top to tail, but you cannot turn it over to fully even out the fillings. This means if you are in bed with a partner who is having the same problem, when you rotate it, you will just be exchanging their body impressions in the mattress (dips), for your own, and these could increase your pain. Maybe you know people who have had a different experience and never had a problem, but this was a constant complaint I had from customers who reported it as a fault and we had to get someone to come out to inspect their mattress. Forewarned is forearmed, and I would much rather tell you this now, than you spend a lot of money on what looks to be a great idea, but in fact could add to your stress.

Now you may think a bed base is not that important, as it is the mattress that you will be lying on, but you would be wrong in making that assumption. The bed base is the foundation of support for your mattress, which in turn supports you. Get this wrong, and the system as a whole could cause you issues. There are two main types of bed bases to choose from, one is a divan base and the other is a bed frame. With a divan base, you can either have a solid base often known a platform top, or a sprung base, and you would buy a separate headboard to either be attached by struts to the bed, or bolt it to the wall above your bed. With a bed frame, you can have straight slats or sprung slats. A bed frame is usually a wooden or metal frame that the mattress sits in, and will take up extra room compared to a divan base, which has the mattress sitting directly on top of it. A bed frame usually comes with a headend, which acts like a headboard but is an integral part of the frame, and either a low-end or high-end footend, although you can sometimes get a frame with no footend, which makes it less intrusive in the room and less likely to cause injury. If your fibromyalgia causes you to bruise easily, and you are tight on space and likely to catch your ankle or bash your leg on a bed frame, don't risk it and get a divan. I know I have caught my leg on a bed frame in a tight space, and it caused me pain and bruising, so I stick with a divan. The benefit of having a divan with a sprung base is it adds more life to the mattress, because it is not hitting against something hard. It also gives a softer feel to the mattress rather than a solid platform top divan base or a bed frame. Even though a sprung slatted bed frame will make the mattress feel softer than a straight slatted bed frame, because there is some give in it, it will still feel firmer than a sprung divan base. So make sure you try the mattress out on a base in the showroom, like you will be getting. So if you try a sprung mattress on a sprung divan base, but you intend to put it on a bed frame, it will feel firmer, and depending on what tension you need for your body weight and height, it may not be good for your pain relief. Something to warn you about, if you have an old base, but you want to put a new mattress on it, especially if it is a sprung base, check for damage to the springs, such as ageing and wear and tear. If you put a new mattress on a base with damaged springs, what do you think is going to happen to the mattress? It will lessen the life of the mattress because it is not being supported by the base, and could in fact damage your new mattress as you start to see it sagging where the springs are damaged underneath. Which means that the mattress will not be fully supportive to the contours of your body and this will result in more fibro pain. This is not a fault with the mattress, but with your base. That's why it's important to usually get a new base, not just a new mattress.

You want look for a bed size that will give you enough space to move around it in. You don't want to be on a small single bed, even as a single person, and feel tight of space. Similarly, if you have a partner, look to get as big as bed as possible, or tell them you need more space and for them to budge up and lie on the edge if need be, and don't feel bad about this, because quality of sleep is important for you, and if they start to touch your pressure points in bed, even if by accident, this will set off your pain and you will have difficulty sleeping. An arm around my neck can set my neck pain off, even though I like that from a partner. If a partner has his legs pressing on some part of my body, say his knee is touching my hip and I am trying to sleep, I can't, my body has to be free. I usually find sleeping in separate beds, or separate houses, a good answer to my pain problem, especially as I like to stay up until the early hours of the night and go to bed when I 'feel' tired. If you are trying to sleep at the same time as your partner, say they like going to bed at 10.30pm, and you like to go to bed at 2.30am, you could be lying in bed for hours, conscious of your pain, trying to sleep. What sort of life is that? What stress is this going to cause you as a result? Will that make you feel good, happy, pleasure? I don't think so!

They say you spend a third of your life in bed, so you can see why it's essential to get the right mattress, divan base or bed frame, and pillows, so you can be as pain free as possible. Remember to pay close attention to your nightwear to make sure it's roomy and comfy enough to not aggravate your pressure points. I have read you can get receding gums with fibromyalgia, or in some cases your teeth can fall out. I have receding gums and I have to ensure I use a sensitive toothpaste for it, so always look after your teeth especially well and floss every night before bed as you don't want those bits of food to get caught anywhere they shouldn't and you have to have dental treatment, as that will be more painful.

KEY POINTS TO REMEMBER

Your sleep problems and related pain problems could be due to the wrong mattress, bed and pillows, not supporting you and relieving your pressure points.

You may need a mattress topper to relieve your pressure points.

You may need a separate bed to your partner or a bigger bed, to prevent your pressure points being touched.

An orthopaedic mattress is not good for a bad back, unless it gives you the right support for your body weight and height. As a general guide, if you are short and slim, you need a softer mattress and bed feel than someone who is taller or larger, as they have a bigger and heavier body mass to support.

Your mattress should come up into the arch of your back to support you. Too firm and you will lie on it like a board, too soft and it will dip down underneath you.

Providing you have the right tension, pocket sprung mattresses tend to be the most supportive spring system, rather than an open coil, because the springs move independently of each other to correctly align your spine.

Always try a mattress out in the showroom on the same type of base as you will be buying, otherwise the feel and tension could be very different from what actually feels comfortable to you and gives you the correct support.

A pillow top mattress may look like a great choice because it adds an extra comfort layer to the mattress, but the fillings will bed down during settlement and often these will cause body impressions to be left in it, which could aggravate fibro pain.

A sprung base can give the mattress a softer feel than a bed frame and adds more life to the mattress.

PART 6
SUPERHERO POWER!

CHAPTER 23
MY BEST KEPT SECRET

Let's examine some of the characteristics of a superhero.

- A freak accident results in the development of the hero's abilities.
- Phenomenal abilities above those of 'normal' humans.
- Exceptional skills.
- Superhuman strength.
- Superpowers.
- Super senses.
- Super intelligent.
- Speed.
- Fearless.
- Courageous.
- Perseverance – Never give up attitude.
- Determined to succeed at whatever they do.
- Motivated by a sense of responsibility and duty.
- Dedicated to their mission.
- Their mind is always thinking.
- A problem solver.
- Confident.
- Kind.
- Considerate.

- Thoughtful.

- Good.

- Respectful.

- Resourceful.

- Hard working.

- A leader.

- Adaptable.

- Creative.

- Organised.

- Efficient.

- A self-starter.

- Knows their own mind.

- Trusts their own instincts.

- Different and quirky.

- An ability to see what others don't.

- A strong moral code, with a willingness to take risks in the name of good, without expecting any reward.

- Secret identity to protect friends and family, often known as an alter ego.

I would like to introduce you to my best-kept secret that no one knew about, until I wrote this book...

FIBRO GIRL TO THE RESCUE!

Fibro Girl is a part of who I am; she is the superhero in me that has superpowers beyond my own physical being. You may call her my alter ego that I created to get me through the physical tough times, because she can do, what I would otherwise tell myself I can't. I particularly allow her to give me super strength when forcing myself to go up a steep cobbled hill into the city centre, a journey I used to make daily to work before I was made redundant and a journey I make now when I walk into the city centre. Sometimes my legs hurt so much from my pelvis joints downwards when walking up that hill, but I like to challenge myself to beat a 'normal' person to the top of it, despite the pain, and then I think to myself, Fibro Girl can do this and say "Fibro Girl to the rescue", and that gives me the super strength, power and momentum, to get up that hill. And guess what? I beat most non-fibro sufferers (as far as I know), to the top of that hill! Go me!! Go Fibro Girl!! I have since discovered other people online who refer to a 'Fibro Girl', but I did not know this when I created her for me, as I previously said, I don't spend as much time in fibro groups like I used to and the bloggers I know who have fibro, never referred to this! So as ACE is the nickname for asexual, and I already told you in Chapter 19, that I am a heteroromantic asexual in sexual orientation; romantically attracted to guys but not sexually, then I like to call myself ACE Fibro Girl. If you ace something it means you excel in it, and now I think I really am Fibro Girl, with those superhuman strengths and abilities, it seems a fitting title.

As I mentioned in a previous chapter, my Grandma always said, "If you don't use it, you lose it", and she was so right. I walked to work for my day job every day and it was at the opposite end of the city to where I live. I don't usually use the buses in my city; I walk everywhere I need to go. I feel better walking, because it keeps my legs moving and makes me feel alive. I want to reiterate what I said in a previous chapter, don't stay indoors in bed, get up and get out and about. If you live alone, being around strangers can make you feel better than being isolated and in pain at home. Getting fresh air and walking can make you feel good. As I mentioned before, I regularly eat mackerel to help my legs be in less pain and stronger and I can sometimes jog or even run part of the way towards the city centre, something I used to do frequently on my way to work – and if you ever want to see something hilarious, it's me, flying up the road with my shopping trolley, I love being different! I regularly use a shopping trolley to carry food shopping home; this ensures that I am not damaging my arms through carrying heavy loads. Pulling a large shopping trolley also keeps my arms nicely toned, and I used to do weightlifting many years ago, so I have bigger than average arm muscles for a girl, giving me more super strength, which I like. If you have not bought a shopping trolley yet, and particularly if you also don't drive, go and get yourself one and save yourself from some pain. A work colleague said to me one morning, she took the bus and then walked and I still got to work faster than her (oh yeah!!!). I am also super fast at walking anyway, even though my legs are one of the most affected areas of my body where my fibro pain is concerned and at times they can feel like they are shaking or jelly-like, but this cannot be seen with the naked eye. I have read that some people with fibro can have their legs collapse, so one thing that I look for in employed work is the ability to sit down at regular intervals which thankfully I could do in my job of 5 years, before I was made redundant. But by being honest about my disability, it is proving extremely difficult to get back into employed work. The truth is, there is a lot of discrimination out there, but I do understand from a manager's point of view why this is, even though it's morally wrong. So I have 19 years retail experience and was in management for 7 of those years. My fibro needs in an employed job are a place to sit down throughout the day, I don't need to sit down every moment of the day, but in-between serving customers I do, or if it's constantly busy then I would need to sit down the majority of the time. I need the toilet on average every hour, I need breaks every two hours due to low blood sugar, to wear trainer socks all the time and not lift above shoulder height. If you can imagine it from an employer's point of view when they recruit, if they have other candidates who do not have these problems, who can be on the shop floor more often and for more hours without a break, who can stand up and theoretically be more productive, who are they going to choose? They overlook the disabled person's attributes, qualities and experience, in favour of this seemingly more productive candidate without any issues. What they don't realise is how hard working and reliable we can be, how much we can be dedicated to the job because we are very grateful and thankful to have one and get out of the house to stop focusing on our pain; how we can be far more experienced and more easily able to build a rapport with customers and close more business. During my redundancy consultation period, I attended a jobs fair, which resulted in a phone call from an agency saying a mobile phone company would like to offer me an interview and could I make that the next day or the day after. I said the day after would be no problem for me, and I want you to know that I have a disability which is fibromyalgia, and I would need to sit down in the job, but I am assuming there would be somewhere to sit down with customers, with it being that type of job. He said he understood my situation from his own family problems with back pain and he thinks there should be a stool there and would that be okay, and I said yes. He said he would phone the shop manager and get back to me, but he did not see a problem. Half an hour later I get a call back to say the manager can't accommodate that, as they have nowhere to sit. I went past that shop on my way home and guess what – oh, they had a lovely tall stool with a chair-like back to it, it was on the customer side, but still, they were talking rubbish. This highlights just how much disabled people can be discriminated against. As the current law stands, according to my Union Rep you cannot take someone to court for discrimination, unless you have been offered a contract of work. I know from experience though, if you are not upfront about your disability, before an offer, it could cause problems if you get the job and they cannot accommodate your reasonable adjustments. The fact you need reasonable adjustments may seem unfair to other team members and if the manager thinks you are too much of a liability or nuisance they may performance manage you out of the job in some other way. They cannot be seen to be doing this because of your disability, as that would be discrimination, but because of your lack of 'capability'. They can make your life so difficult that you want to leave, and to be honest it's not worth the stress and anxiety that such a situation would cause you and increase your fibro pain so much so, that it could be debilitating. So it's always best to be honest. I was an honest manager but not everyone is and a lot of bullying can go on in the workplace. I say this not to depress you, but because I understand your plight and what you are up against. If you are in an employed job, make sure you are part of a Union so you have extra protection should the worst happen. A Union Rep can give you advice about work law and can attend meetings with your employers should they need to, in regard to things like disciplinaries, and constructive or unfair dismissal cases. I am a member of USDAW and my membership provides other benefits such as accident cover both in work and out of work.

In the job I was made redundant from which I enjoyed, I was the only fitted bedroom specialist in a large department store, I was required to approach customers, build a rapport with them, talk to them about the free no obligation design service we offered, demonstrate the products with features and benefits, and match their needs to those, then book them a free no-obligation design service appointment or get them a brochure sent out. I was only allowed to sit down because I have fibro; otherwise it was against the rules. I got to go to the toilet whenever I wanted in-between serving customers; I had breaks every 2 hours; I wore trainer socks all year round, which was only allowed because I have fibro and I had no heavy lifting, and I was often a top performer in the country for percentage of sales over target, but sadly I had to leave, even though I had growth for my performance every year, because the overall costs of the business were too high and they reduced the hours to part-time. However, I do believe everything happens for a reason and it's important to look at redundancy as the opportunity of a lifetime to pursue your dreams, passions, missions and life goals, so that is what I am doing and I am super excited about that. With fibro, it's essential not to panic in these situations as you don't want to instil fear, anxiety and worry into your mind, because you know it will increase your fibro pain and flare ups, and then you will be in no position to apply for other jobs or pursue your dreams, as you will be too sick. Just keep reminding yourself of all of your positive qualities and strengths about yourself and focus on other stuff, besides the urgency to get money coming in.

Remember we have just discussed the qualities of a superhero, now I want you to go and grab a pen and paper and write down how many of those qualities you have, be honest and don't be modest. This is about recognising your many strengths. Remember, it is our 'freak accident' of having fibro, that makes us have superhuman strengths and abilities of being able to cope, manage, and stay strong, despite the pain, so that is one quality that encompasses many to start you off. Now go!!

By now, you should have a list of positives about you, because of both yourself and your fibro. This is great in starting to see the benefits and blessings of fibro. If we go around hating our fibro, we are essentially hating a huge part of our self and that is no good as we need to self-love and care for our self deeply, we need to accept it and the strengths it gives us, otherwise, we are forced to have more pain because of that negative emotion in our body.

I recognise my own superhero qualities, not just when Fibro Girl is around, but because of the way I manage my fibromyalgia using the power of my mind to block out a lot of the pain, it means I can do far more than some people with fibro can and I am grateful for that. And because I have studied personal and professional development since 2012, I am far more intelligent and experienced in the right things than I ever used to be; accessing far more than 10% of my brain, it's like being in another world entirely and having lots of superpowers, strengths, abilities and skills, that I never dreamt I could possibly possess! Which is a huge difference from the depressed girl I was before 2012! Who lacked self-confidence; strength and self-love; self-worth; and felt like dying and what's the point to life! Nowadays, I love living and want to live to be at least 100, and thanks to having all those superhero qualities, I know it's possible! A superhero can make the impossible; possible, so never forget you can do that too. Be your own superhero and take the world by storm!

KEY POINTS TO REMEMBER

Develop a superhero mindset.

Believe your fibro gives you superhero abilities.

Fibro Girl is your alter ego you can use to get you through tough times and to challenge yourself. Use her to do something that as yourself you could not do, but as superhero Fibro Girl you could, because she gives you that superhero strength and you know if Fibro Girl can do it then so can you.

Say "Fibro Girl to the rescue", for that boost of strength when facing difficulties. Think of her coming along and getting you through whatever it is that you are facing.

Be your own superhero and recognise those superhero qualities you have, when Fibro Girl is NOT around.

CHAPTER 24

21ST MINDSET WITH A TEENAGER LIFESTYLE AND A ROCKSTAR ATTITUDE!

To quote Henry Ford, *"Whether you think you can or you think you can't, you're right".*

To quote Les Brown, *"You have greatness within you."*

I have a 21st mindset, in other words, my mindset is that of a 21 year old. My birth certificate age is just that, it does not have any bearing on my current life or lifestyle. When I was younger in birth certificate age, I was older, I even looked older, now I am older in birth certificate age; I am younger. You have choices in life and you can choose to be any age you want in your mind. What you think, you become, thus you can create your own reality based on a younger age, should you choose to. This is how you become and stay young, naturally, without plastic surgery or Botox. So this means, I believe I can do anything a 21 year old can do, if I want to, and this mindset works really well with my teenager lifestyle. This means I do young stuff; watch young stuff; listen to young music; wear young brands; live in a young environment; have younger friends; get attracted to younger guys and have a lot in common with them, and can potentially can have a younger boyfriend. A lot of my online friends are in their early to mid twenties and some of my in person guy friends are too. So despite having fibromyalgia, in 2017 I went clubbing to a Ministry Of Sound event and I go out clubbing now sometimes too. I love dancing and don't let my fibro stop me from doing that. I adore going to theme parks as often as possible, I go to places like Shrek Adventureland in London, and zoos and aquariums. I listen to dance, club, pop, and techno music the most. I watch super-hero movies and Disney and Pixar films, and in 2017 I went to Disneyland Paris for my 21st mindset birthday celebration, complete with 21st birthday banners, 21st birthday confetti and balloons, and a 21st card. I had a Toy Story room that I adored. I get bored very easily, just like a 15 year old, and I am a lights, camera, action, noise, and doing person. So whilst a lot of people with the same birth certificate age as me, (which is just over 4 decades, and is completely irrelevant to who I am, as it's not reflective of the real me), seem to be happy to stay at home watching TV, to have peace and quiet, adopt a slow pace of life, like going out in nature looking at scenery and historical buildings, watching the news and such, all of that bores me. I want to do young, fun stuff. I like noise, hustle and bustle. I like to live a vibrant teenager lifestyle, one that is energetic and fills me with excitement and magic. Life is for living to the max, 24/7. I like to be active and doing stuff all the time. Going out and having fun as much as possible and at other times vlogging, blogging, and learning more personal and professional development stuff, so I can improve myself and my life. I love a teenager style relationship, without the sex, but with plenty of kissing, cuddling, going out on dates together, and feeling loved up 24/7. This is how you stay young, like a superhero rockstar!

I am an unconventional, non-traditional, un-stereotypical female. I hate washing up, cooking and cleaning, and just do the bare minimum I can to get by and I mean minimum. Apart from dusting the TV and around the TV when I occasionally switch it on to watch a movie on Blu-ray or DVD, I don't do dusting. I have a rockstar attitude where housework is concerned; I don't sweat the small stuff. Why go to all that pain by getting up a ladder to dust as it will only get dusty again and no one is going to see the tops of your wardrobes or shelves anyway? Don't waste your precious life on things like this that don't matter. A rockstar does not care about house-work, they are too busy having fun and enjoying their life and their time, working their mission, developing themselves, pleasing their audience and following their dreams. They are too busy perform-ing to work in the kitchen, they will eat out or get a takeaway with throwaway cutlery, or have someone make their meals for them, and this is a great attitude to have if you have fibro. Fibromyalgia can zap your energy, being in constant pain can be very energy draining so I don't want you to spend your life doing menial tasks that don't really matter to your happiness. Find ways of putting you first and reducing the amount of time you spend on house-work. The last thing you want to do is to be stood up over a kitch-en sink washing up, if your legs and body are in pain. This applies to other household tasks. I don't hoover everyday, I hoover when I think it is necessary and I don't iron my clothes until I need to wear them and I try to get as many non-iron clothes as possible. I never iron bed linen anymore, as I am just going to get it crumpled again when I sleep in it, so what is the point in doing this? People waste so much time on housework, when mostly it is just them seeing the end result, unless you enjoy housework, it's just a point-less waste of precious life and energy. If you have fibro, you need to conserve your energy for enjoyable things and doing things that encourage you to get your feel good factor antidotes every single day of your life. Like a rockstar, think life should be one big party from beginning to end, every single day of your life and strive for that feeling as much as possible by taking action to achieve it.

I have noticed that those who have fibro and have a husband and kids to look after, have far less energy and more pain, as they are busy taking care of others and expelling their precious energy on others and not themselves. I think if they spent more time having fun, doing what makes them feel good and alive, and not doing housework for others, they would have far less pain and a better quality of life. So if that is your situation, why not say something and start living your life for you? The clock is ticking. I am not interested in cooking or cleaning for a guy and expect him to be able to look after himself, just like I can look after myself. When dating and in terms of a potential relationship, I set boundaries in place early on, that he can buy his own food to cook or eat and that I don't do housework for a guy as it takes me all my time and energy to look after myself and to lead a young, fun, and energetic life. I use paper plates to save on washing up, and Jane Asher non-stick Silicone Liners that are usually used in cake tins, I line with tin foil, (or greaseproof paper – which is meant to be a better option due to the health concerns associated with metals), to put in the oven, in place of using and washing up a grill pan. Any other washing up I save to do in one go, and block time out for it. This means I don't have to waste 5 nights in pain at the sink, instead, I can just spend an hour and a half one day and get it done in one go. For safety reasons, you have to be mindful of the temperature you use these liners at because they can burn and never leave them in the oven for longer than they need, or ever go out and leave them, because you don't want a fire. So if you haven't got a dishwasher, or if it pains you to fill that, either get your other half or the kids to do more washing up and housework, or try using paper plates and cutlery you can throw away. You could use plastic cups too that you should be able to recycle, and foil baking trays you can throw away. Do not feel ashamed of reducing things that cause you pain and increasing things that make you happier, because you are worth it. I don't live with my parents, but my mum gets horrified when I say I leave the washing up to do in one go, do I care, no, she likes being a housewife and I don't. She likes doing housework – I don't! I live on my own so I can please myself what I do. If anyone does not like what I do, they are welcome to come and do it for me

– it is their choice! My choice is to live life my way, and not worry about such things. If I spent time each night doing that, it would zap my energy to do stuff that is far more rewarding and productive to me. I don't spend much time in my kitchen, so out of sight, mostly out of mind, until I run out of cutlery! – As I prefer to use real ones of those as opposed to plastic at the moment. It is also more economical to use less water by doing washing up in one go and you can just squirt washing up liquid in bowls and rinse to get the bulk of food deposits off if you need to.

I also sometimes buy pre-prepared salads in plastic bowls that I can just throw away in the recycling bin after I have eaten its contents. But be very careful of these, because I started to feel more tired and lacking in energy, with headaches for a number of months, not realising that my local supermarket had added sugar to the ingredients of their "Sweet and Crunchy Salad". Even though it had sweetcorn added to it, to make it sweet. As I said previously, I am allergic to sugar, I am okay with 'most' natural sugars, I say most because I can't have honey as it's too sugary for me. So added sugar is a huge no, no for me. I always have some side effects from eating it. It can make me feel dizzy, in the worse case scenario like the room is spinning around and I am on a ship in rough seas; very tired, lethargic, lacking in energy with a need to sleep, and tightness in my head, and I never thought a salad would have that added to it, so be sure to check the ingredients of everything you buy. If you think you have ongoing fibro fog and you get headaches and can't think clearly, and lack in energy, and always feel tired, it may not be your fibro that is causing you that problem, but sugar, or another food. So go and get checked by a qualified homeopath for food allergies. That is how I found out about all my allergies. My own doctor said he would only ever test me for wheat, not anything else, and those patch tests are not always 100% accurate, and as I already knew I was allergic to wheat, he said if the test came back negative for it, I would still continue not to eat it anyway, wouldn't I? And I said yes.

Another thing that is great to have is a living apart together relationship. This means you are in an intimate relationship with your partner, but you live in separate places. That way you can arrange your life, lifestyle, and environment, to give you the most energy. You can do the least amount of housework and things that cause you pain, and do what makes you feel good, without the worry of what a partner will think and feel. As most people argue over money in a relationship, if you live in separate places and don't share household bills, you won't have this stress that your pain could do without. You can still be married and have this arrangement too.

KEY POINTS TO REMEMBER

You have choices in life and you can choose to be any age you want in your mind and lifestyle.

What you think, you become, thus you can create your own reality based on a younger age, should you choose to.

Unless you enjoy housework, it's just a pointless waste of precious life and energy. Find ways of putting you first and reducing the amount of time you spend on housework

Save time on washing up by using paper plates and cutlery or get other people in your household to do it for you.

Consider a Living Apart Together arrangement (LAT) so you don't have to worry about a partner and can live a more stress free life to reduce your pain.

CHAPTER 25
SUPERHERO ROCKSTAR FIBRO
GIRL POWER!

By now you should have read the tips throughout this book to lower your fibro pain and make you live an extraordinary fibro life. If you haven't and you just skim read this book, then go back to the beginning and start over. Remember to dip in and out of it whenever you are focusing on a particular aspect of your life that you need to improve to decrease your pain. Pay close attention to the Key Points for quick reference. If you just bought this book and skipped to the back page, you will be pleased to know that I am about to write an overview of the book with a list of each aspect of your life that you need to address to increase that feel good factor and decrease your pain, with 'Quick Fixes' in a number of these areas. You still need to read the whole book, for in-depth knowledge of how to reduce your fibro pain, have more energy and feel happier. If you take your pain seriously and value the quality of your life, you will not only read this book from cover to cover, you will take action and do the hard work it takes to change your life, for the better, forever. Nothing in this book will work, unless you commit to taking action and make positive changes in your life. Words are just words, until you give them meaning and make them a reality, through continued application and persistent action.

Having a positive mindset is absolutely crucial to decreasing your fibro pain. Most people look at their fibro pain and think and believe they are 'suffering', but if you think you are suffering then you will, you have it for life, so never be a victim of it.

Without a positive mindset, you will keep focusing on your pain, which in turn will make you feel unhappy and lethargic. What we focus on expands, the more we think about our pain; the more pain we will receive. The more pain we receive, the unhappier we become, the unhappier we become, the more our energy depletes. So don't put your life on hold and wait for some magic outside cure to fix you, be a superhero to yourself and save yourself from pain.

You have a choice, you can choose to be a sufferer or you can choose to be a Fibro Girl, with a warrior-like rockstar attitude and a 21st mindset, with an ability to block out a lot of the pain using the power of your mind to be consciously unaware of it. Choice is power, making a decision is power, so choose to decide to never be a victim of your fibro but to manage it like a "Superhero Rockstar", to have less pain, more energy and feel happier. Use fibro to your advantage. Use it to look after yourself better than ever before, to literally reflect upon your life and all the major aspects of it, to see how you can improve your life to decrease your stress, anxiety and worry, and get more good, happiness, pleasure, feeling safe and loved, and having faith in your life, to decrease your pain. Make it your mission to do this every day and see how your quality of life can improve.

These are the 25 aspects of your life that you need to examine as causes of your fibro pain and how you are going to decrease it.

1) Body.

2) Mind and mindset.

3) Foods you eat.

4) Medications you take.

5) Shopping.

6) Housework.

7) Clothes.

8) Attitude.

9) Thoughts.

10) Feelings.

11) Emotions.

12) Spirit/soul.

13) Intuition.

14) Mission, goals, ambitions and dreams.

15) Career/job

16) Lifestyle.

17) Weather.

18) Sleep.

19) Environment.

20) Hobbies.

21) Finances.

22) Friends and Family.

23) Relationship with yourself.

24) Relationship with others.

25) Love, intimacy and sex.

Let's recap on what it's like to be a rockstar, so you can apply this way of living and these character traits to your fibro life to reduce your pain.

Rockstars don't get much sleep and can live on less sleep and still perform well. They have a ton of energy and they use music to energise themselves. They buy quick and easy foods to eat, eat out, or get someone to make it for them. They don't sweat the small stuff. They have a sense of humour and don't take life too seriously. If they make mistakes (think of fibro fog), they accept it, it does not stop them performing and they carry on. If they hurt themselves and are in physical pain they don't moan about it, they accept it as part of their life. They don't give into pain, but rather use it as a tool to challenge themselves, and they work harder to achieve their end result; their goals, ambitions and dreams, and continue to give the performance of their life. They are not a victim of circumstance, but a leader of their life. They will always try to be the last one standing. They have a warrior-like attitude and always want to be top of their game and will let nothing stop them from giving that rockstar performance to leave fans feeling energised and breathless.

Rockstars don't worry about creating a mess; they are more concerned with living life to the max and living their life with passion and meaning. They play to their strengths and stick to what they are good at and excel in, practicing their craft over and over again to perfect it, whilst having the flexibility and adaptability to make changes whenever necessary to cope with any challenge life throws at them and to continuously develop themselves.

Rockstars are:

- Focused.

- Knowledgeable.

- Intentional.

- Great at managing their time.

- Organised.

- Can look after themselves.

- They love performing so much, and don't let any pain or frustration stop them.

- They know when to take time out for them, to recharge and re-energise themselves to give an even better performance of their life.

Let's recap on what mindset and lifestyle you need to reduce your conscious fibro pain.

- Block out your pain in your mind, don't think about it and pay no attention to it.

- Distract your mind and do things to take your mind off it.

- Consciously make a pain free space in your subconscious where your soul and being live, and focus your life on that part of your mind, rather than focusing on your body pain.

- Adopt a teenage lifestyle and environment.

- Have a 21st mindset. Think young, be young; act young.

To have a 21st mindset you need to think, 'I can do anything a 21 year old can do because my mind tells me so'. If you focus on your body pain, you won't be able to, as you will be focusing on negative energy, lack and can't, when you need to focus on what you actually want to do, think you can do, and do it. You have to literally think, 'I can do this, because I am 21 and this is what a 21 year old would do. No ifs, no buts and no maybes. That's it. If they can do it then so can I'. Think of the positive outcome, how great you will feel, and hold onto that feeling, and take action. Do not let any doubt come into your mind because of your fibro. Know you can deal with any outcome, and make the gain greater than any potential pain and you will achieve far more in your life. Remember this quote; "When the gain is greater than the pain, you will do it, when the pain is greater than the gain, you won't!" For me, the pain of the fear of not being able to walk in the future and having regrets that I did not live my life to the max, is far higher than the pain I get from making myself walk up a hill to go into the city centre. My mum tells me about people she meets at the hospital when she is going for her usual tests; who have fibro and are on crutches. She informs me of when she hears of people who have fibro and are bed ridden or in a wheelchair, and I realise how very lucky and fortunate I am, and how I will do everything within my power to ensure I never get to that stage. Fibro can get worse, but I am not going to dwell on that, 'can', does not mean it will, and there are people who 'claim' to have 'cured' themselves from fibro, so never give up hope.

Don't be driven by the fear of pain, but by the fear of not being able to walk and living your life with regrets. This is what pushes me to do the things I do, to be bold and to be brave. If you are in a wheelchair, don't live in fear of it; live in fear of what will happen if you don't put energy and effort into other things and you let your mind become sluggish and inactive! If you are on crutches or in a wheelchair you can still adapt your life using the power of your mind to achieve amazing things. The problem with being in a wheelchair is you lose the strength of those muscles that allow you to stand up, but that does not mean to say you cannot retrain yourself to use those again, nor should you accept it as a problem that stops you from living life to the full. Remember that guy I mentioned earlier in the beginning of this book, Nick Vijucic? No Arms. No Legs. NO LIMITS? He does not let his limits limit him and neither should you!

Whatever your physical condition, to block out pain you need make the conscious decision to become consciously unaware of it by creating a pocket of your mind that is reserved for your soul and free from the direct effects of fibro. It should be where your inner child lives; your core being; and you. Have a pain threshold in your mind, for normal, everyday, permanent fibro pain, and when you have extra pain on top of that, that is when it will become conscious and you will be able to work out what you did differently from your normal routine that increased your pain, so you can determine the aggravator and reduce or get rid of it from your life. This could be related to any of those 25 aspects of your life mentioned at the beginning of this chapter and detailed throughout this book.

If you are the type of person that can't usually sleep if you go to bed before midnight, then know that is okay, because a 21 year old will often be up until the early hours, that is normal for a 21 year old and you are 21. And don't care what others think, live your life for you, not them.

QUICK FIXES

Your fibro pain and lack of energy are directly related to your internal and external environments, which is why it is so important you re-read this book thoroughly and take action to change your life. Let's recap on some of the things you can do right now to reduce your fibro pain and live a better quality of life.

Food:

Make eating mackerel a must. Eat it daily for maximum benefit of the high level of omega 3 oil it contains. This is one of the most important changes you can make to your diet to reduce your fibro pain. Your legs desperately need that oil to ease movement and pain. Don't think about it, just do it, and see the huge difference it can make to your body and life.

Cut out all refined sugars; fruit juice and fruit are okay. Cut out alcohol, which is full of sugar and fermented, so it encourages candida overgrowth, which is the most common cause of fungal infection in humans and will add to your body discomfort and therefore increase your pain and deplete your energy. Cut out wheat and gluten. Wheat encourages candida overgrowth in the gut in particular. Then try cutting out yeast and dairy; yeast is another one that encourages candida overgrowth. You can still treat yourself to sugar free, wheat free, gluten free, chocolate and ice cream once in a while from an independent health shop. Monitor your carb intake to see if certain carbs make you feel tired and in pain, so you can adjust your diet to have less of those, or cut them completely if you are able to. If you have low blood sugar, you will usually always need to have some carbs, so consult a doctor or qualified nutritionist about this.

Cut out normal size tomatoes that act like aspirin on the stomach, and cut out mushrooms, grapes, cheese and all yoghurt, which can encourage candida overgrowth too.

Take a supplement in liquid format that has billions of good bugs such as Hylak. It may be preserved in alcohol and this is acceptable because it stops them dying off but otherwise you should not drink alcohol because of the sugar and fermentation aspects of it and some alcohols contain wheat and gluten.

Drink:

I already mentioned cutting out alcohol completely. Remember, you have a 21 year old mindset and live like a teenager and kids have no fear, so you don't need alcohol to do crazy things, you can happily enjoy your crazy times consciously and be so proud you have no fear, you can rid yourself of your inhibitions, and get high on fruit juice and life, believe me, I do this, and it is possible. It actually makes you stronger and able to do what others can't – superpower. I can be out clubbing until the very end at 2am or 3am, and still be dancing even though I have fibro, whereas some guys younger than me in birth certificate age, such as 18 year olds, can't hack the pace.

Get rid of caffeine drinks and fizzy drinks that have sugar, and replace with herbal teas. Use chamomile, 3 ginger, and liquorice.

Replace dairy milk with lactose free milk or soya milk, if you are not allergic to these.

Medications:

Ask if they are helping you, are they working? Are they causing you any side effects? Are you in more pain since you started taking meds for your fibro? I don't take any meds for fibro. The pharmaceutical industry is big business and it pays them to get you to take pills. Often you need one pill to counteract the effects of another, who is this helping, you or the pharmaceutical industry? Always consult your doctor or medical health professional before changing medications or coming off them.

Clothes:

To stop your feet from swelling, don't wear 'normal' socks, wear trainer socks with ventilation panels all year round, including throughout winter, and wear only memory foam slippers. Buy practical footwear, that have supportive insoles, not shoes that squash your toes, have a high heel and flimsy insoles.

If your tummy is sensitive to having pressure on it, wear loose fitting clothing, such as loose fitting PJs and trousers. Get the next size up if it helps you to be in less pain.

Sleep:

Sleep when you feel tired and not when society dictates you should go to sleep. If you are a night owl and would rather be up until the early hours and go to sleep in the late morning or day, then do that. Embrace your natural sleep pattern.

Your bed can cause you pain. Unless you are tall or big in body mass, an orthopaedic mattress will not usually help with back pain and can make it worse. Even then, you need get the right tension for you. Get rid of your open coil mattress and go for a latex or pocket sprung bed that is supportive and correctly aligns the spine in a tension that is right for your body weight and height. If you lie on the mattress, it should come up to support your spine, not be like a board and too hard for you, or too soft and dipping down underneath you. If you need your mattress to have a softer feel on top because of your pressure points, get a mattress topper. Use a waterproof mattress protector and get rid of feather or down pillows and use one latex pillow instead.

Housework:

To save energy and stop being in so much pain, cut down on the amount of housework you do and get your family or your spouse to cook for themselves and do their share or more of the housework!

If you don't have a dishwasher, use paper plates you can throw away to save you from washing up. Use silicone cake liners and line them with tin foil or greaseproof paper, instead of using a grill pan, to save you from washing that up. For safety be mindful of the temperature you use these at as they can burn and you don't want a fire. Another alternative is to use foil containers that you can put in the oven and throw away after use. Although there are health concerns around using aluminium in your cooking materials and equipment, so you can Google 'aluminium health concerns', to find out about that and make your own mind up. I have an iron sauce-pan for that reason, although now I eat all my vegetables raw, I don't use a pan, to save myself some washing up. Get ready made salads so you can throw away packaging and save on washing up. Be sure to check the ingredients first. Store your washing up to do in one go to reduce your pain standing at the sink and to make more time for fun stuff!

If you can't see it, or it's up high near your ceiling, don't dust it, unless you have dust allergies or enjoy dusting.

Hoover only when you need to, not every day if you don't have to.

Only iron clothes that need it, which is when you are actually going to wear them. Buy non-iron clothes as much as possible. Stop ironing bed linen; it's only going to get crumpled again.

Relationships with others:

Hang around and talk with people who make you feel good about yourself, who are like-minded, who understand you, and who speak positively and support you in your goals, ambitions and dreams. Avoid people who are regularly negative, who are unsupportive, who have a victim mentality and permanently in 'suffer syndrome', cut them out of your life or limit the time you spend with them.

Relationship with yourself/self-love:

Use positive self-talk on a daily and consistent basis and think positively, to counteract those negative emotions, which creates bad energy in your body and ignites your pain. Praise yourself and give yourself credit for what you have achieved so far in your life! Write down a minimum of 10 things you like about yourself and refer to that daily. Every morning, say out loud the things that you are grateful for, followed by your antidote affirmations in this book, that you type out or hand write, and read them every day forever, ideally while looking in the mirror. Allow at least 21 days to set them as a good habit, as it takes 21 days to form a new habit. Write down 5 successes at the end of every day, however big or small, even if you just managed to take the rubbish out or had a shower and got dressed. Small wins should always be celebrated as well as big ones.

Change what you consume:

What you consume directly impacts your thoughts, feelings and emotions, which in turn drives what actions you do or don't take and what decisions you make.

Stop listening to, reading, and watching, negative stuff. Stop watching the news; it is full of negativity about murder, death and rape. Stop watching endless hours of TV that is designed to get you hooked on the drama and emotions of negative storylines and does not stretch or grow you in any way to be the best version of you that there can be. Start watching motivational and inspiration videos and reading motivational and inspirational books and getting into personal and professional development.

Change your state:

Change your state through what you consume, through movement and music. If you lack energy on a consistent basis, you need to work on altering your lifestyle and mindset; change your focus; yourself; the people you surround yourself with; your environments, and your life.

Your goals, ambitions and dreams:

You need to have a life purpose and know why you are here on this earth to have hope for the future, to be and stay motivated, which will help to create positive energy. Everyone has a life purpose and if you don't know what this is, make it your mission to obtain it. You being born is a miracle and you only have a certain time on this earth so you need to make the most of it, to live your life with no regrets and leave your mark on this world in an impactful way. If you have nothing to look forward to, that will zap your energy as you will have little hope for the future and your life will stagnate. Fill your life up with things that inspire you; enlighten you; delight you; make you progress in some way, and that grow and stretch you. Take a course, pursue a passion, and get a hobby. If you work towards something meaningful, it will take your mind off your pain and give you a reason to get out of bed in the morning. It will make you lead a more fulfilling and vibrant life, so you truly feel like you are thriving and not just surviving.

WHAT HAPPENS NEXT?

Some people will read this book from cover to cover and find it an incredibly helpful and useful tool to reduce their fibro pain. They will see nuggets of information and they will apply those specific nuggets and achieve some improvement in their life, I hope this applies to you. The odd few may take it completely to heart and really love this stuff, take action, and see a vast difference and improvement in their life, and I hope this person is definitely you! And some people will read through this book, they will look at it and they will say, "but my circumstances are nothing like hers and she does not know the extent of my pain, it's easy for her to say all this, it won't work for me, it's rubbish," and so they take no action. They try to get to sleep at a 'reasonable' hour on a mattress that is unsuitable for their condition, and when they eventually get to sleep, an hour and a half later if they are lucky, they wake up feeling un-refreshed, in more pain, and their legs are heavy and jelly-like all at once, yet they stay in bed feeling that pain, trying to get more rest. They post on Facebook 'you don't know what it's like to 'suffer' with this illness', to show the world how much suffering they are under and how they are a victim of this illness. They take their meds as the doctor told them to do, despite the fact their pain is no better, they hang around with people who agree with them about their pain and how awful it is we suffer like this, they do the usual housework that is expected of them, they live the age they are, and the lifestyle that conventionally goes with that, and they repeatedly say things like, "when I was young", and "when you get to my age", or "when you get to a certain age", not acknowledging the fact they have choices in life, they can choose to be any age they want to be, to live any lifestyle they choose; they can choose to manage fibromyalgia like a Superhero Rockstar or they can choose to put this book down and never look at it again. I hope this isn't you. Let me ask you a question, what have you got to lose by trying some of the things I teach in this book? And what will happen if you don't? Will the fear of failure and of trying new things outweigh your fibro pain so you decide it's not worth trying? Or will the fear of the consequences of what might happen if you don't try some of this stuff, win the day? What type of person are you? And what type of person do you want to become? Will you be a robot and powerless, or a leader of your own life? Being fearless is about facing your fears head on, going through those fears and learning lessons along the way. I know it's super tough, but you can be your own superhero, you have the superpower to change your life, in fact you were always the only one who had that superpower given to you from birth, it's your birth right, so why aren't you using it? It has only your name on it.

Remember to go back to the beginning of this chapter and look at all 25 aspects of your life and read this book again to see how you can improve your life and reduce your pain in all those areas, feel free to add your own ideas as you unleash your fibro girl inside of you and get those superpowers and super senses and abilities working for you. I know you never thought you could possibly possess these, but believe me you do, so unleash your fibro girl; your 21st mindset; your teenager lifestyle, and take the world by storm. Be your own superhero and never let your limits limit you, live your life for you with no regrets, but full of everything that gives you your antidotes to ease your pain!

Remember this quote and live by it every single day of your life: *"Feeling good is the antidote to feeling bad. Feeling pleasure is the antidote to feeling pain. Feeling happy is the antidote to feeling sad. Feeling safe; loved and having faith, is the antidote to feeling fear."*

Write the following antidote affirmations on post-it notes:

Today I feel good.

Today I feel pleasure.

Today I feel happy.

Today I feel safe.

Today I feel loved.

Today I have faith.

Put these post-it notes around your home and especially next to your mirrors and read them out loud every day, at least 3 times a day, forever. This will help re-wire your mind for positive thinking.

This book should help you eliminate stuff that makes you feel bad and add stuff that makes you feel good, energised, happier, and in less pain. You have the power to make it happen and turn your life around, with the right tools, I believe in you. I was depressed for years before having fibro and I thought there was no way out, but I overcame it in 2012 because I got fibromyalgia and knew I could not allow myself to have a negative mindset anymore, and so I know anything is possible.

It's hard changing your life, but you must if you want to reduce your fibro pain and lead a happier and better quality of life in spite of having fibro, and in many ways because of it. You have to change your mindset to a positive one, with a - I can do what I like - regardless of fibro attitude. Notice I said what you like, not what others want, but you. If doing things for another person doesn't make you happy, gives you more pain, and zaps your energy, don't do it. You have to stop caring about what other people think, including those closest to you, they aren't you and they don't have your condition, so they can't stop your pain or reduce it, you need to assert yourself and tell them, "this is the way things are now, if you want to work with me great, this is what I need". Stop 'acting your age' and doings things that don't make you feel happy; good; safe; give you pleasure, make you feel loved or have faith, and stop being restricted by limiting beliefs that are keeping your pain locked inside of you.

Change is difficult and uncomfortable, because you have been a product of conditioning since birth. You have been taught to rely on others for your food and drink, for your education, for your medication, for knowing right from wrong, for formulating habits and ways of thinking that are not your own, they are not in keeping with your inner being and soul and you have been swept up in them. You have been taught how you should look, what you should wear, who and what you should find attractive, how you should have your hair, what interests and hobbies to have, what people you should hang around with, what 9-5 job you should get, and how you should live your life day-to-day. You have had fear instilled into you through the media, from those closest to you, from strangers, from doctors and medical practitioners and from yourself. The amount of counselling I've had in the past is immense. I had years of it on and off. I had CBT (cognitive behavioural therapy), CAT (cognitive analytical therapy), I was even diagnosed with GAD (Generalised Anxiety Disorder level 4, years ago), which I had to work hard to manage and reduce in intensity. It wasn't until I started personal and professional development in 2012, that I really started to see a dramatic shift in myself and my life and I finally got to see the good in me as I am. I started to believe in my abilities and myself; I started to learn things that would develop and grow me more as a person. I started to stop needing others to help me change my life and I started to do the work to change it for myself. I started to see there was far more to life than I had ever been taught and the only reason I needed these other people in my life –

the counsellors and therapists; was because I felt there was some-thing wrong with my life and me. There was something wrong with my life; that was true; it was me that was wrong for me, be-cause I was not leading the right life for me and I had disempower-ing beliefs. I did not believe in myself, I did not see good qualities in my life or me, I did not have any support from others, but I did not have support from me. I was looking for answers from those who have been conditioned themselves. I was listening to the way I should be, not the unique way that is good for unique me. So ask yourself; am I different? Do I want to be different? Or do I want to fit in and be like others and just lead a 'normal' life? I hate to break it to you, but there is no such thing as a 'normal' life and especially where fibromyalgia is concerned. You have to accept that fibrom-yalgia has changed your life and so that means you have to change your life to adapt to it and thrive within it. You have to know it is not your fault, you did not know about this conditioning, but now you do know, to ignore it would be deeply hurtful to yourself. In a time when right now you feel powerless and that you have no con-trol over your pain and how it makes you feel, I am telling you, you do. You have the power of choice. You have to find purpose and meaning in every day and you have to consciously and coura-geously stop being a product of conditioning and start living for you as the fibro girl – or guy, you were always born to be!

If your fibro meds are not reducing your pain, why are you still taking them? When you go to the doctors for yet another pill, what are you hoping to achieve from that? Are you hoping for a cure? As of yet, as I write this book, there is no official cure for fibromyalgia and you have it for life. The doctor cannot cure you; they are trying to help ease your symptoms. Instead of medicating, why not go through this book again and learn how to remove as much negativ-ity and bad stuff from your life as possible and start to live again, start to laugh again, start to have fun again, and live as youthful you. Go get friends that inspire you and make you feel happy and good. If you are housebound, go on online forums that are empowering, inspirational, and happy. Start doing blogging and get your own tribe. You can start a free blog at www.wordpress.com. I have been blogging for almost 9 years and it has changed my life. When I first started to blog, my confidence increased, I grew happier, and I felt in control of something in a time in my life when I felt out of control.

You have to believe it when I say, you do have the power to change your life and turn it around; in fact you are your only guarantee of doing that, the answers lie within you. If you are relying on others for your own happiness, and that includes waiting for a cure from fibromyalgia, you are giving away your personal power and that means you will be and stay powerless. It's hard to hear that nothing and no one can change your life but you, especially when you are in so much pain and struggle, but you don't have to be. Master your mind to learn to see things differently – go back through this book to see just how to do that. You can choose to stay a victim of your fibro and of your life to date, or you can choose to take charge of your life and your fibro, right now, and be a master of them. You can choose to own your fibro and your life, or you can choose to allow your fibro pain to own you and keep reacting to what comes your way in life. Think of fibro as giving you a new lease of life, not taking your life away from you, but giving you an opportunity to get a happier, more fulfilling and fun life for you, that is quirky and different, because if you don't, it will hurt you more. Fibro forces you to be happy!

Understand how beautiful, wonderful and amazing you are, in your own right. Believe that everything happens for a reason, that your fibro makes you stronger and you deserve and are worthy of living, a superhero rockstar life.

By following what I teach in this book, by mastering all of your internal and external environments using those 6 antidotes in a disciplined way, day in, day out, you can reduce the pain yourself. It will take lot of hard work and discipline on your part; it will require strength when you feel you have no more. But you owe it to yourself, to stop looking for answers outside of you and start looking for answers from within you. You can do it, you can be your own superhero and save yourself from pain, I believe in you and I am rooting for you.

I hope you have learnt some things from this Quirky Book and even if you just take one thing from this book, know your fibro does not own you, and you are stronger because of it.

If you have enjoyed reading this book, please like <u>ACE FIBRO GIRL</u> on Facebook at <u>www.facebook.com/acefibrogirl</u> and leave an honest review on that page and Amazon.

PERSONAL POWER DECLARATIONS

Remember to put into practice on a daily basis, saying these affirmations as your personal power declarations, out loud every morning when you wake up, and throughout the day to keep topped up on positivity, to keep your mindset in a good state, and keep pain levels to a minimum. They work best if you say them in front of the mirror and put your hand on your heart at the same time. Write them down on post-it notes and put these next to all the mirrors in your home, as well as around your home in places they are likely to catch your eye and you feel compelled to read them.

"I OWN MY FIBRO; IT DOES NOT OWN ME. I AM IN CONTROL; I FEEL MY POWER AND MY ENERGY."

"Today I feel Good. Today I feel Pleasure. Today I feel Happy. Today I feel Safe. Today I feel Loved. Today I have Faith".

Whenever times get difficult and you feel you can't climb that hill, or walk that far, or move a certain way, but you need to, say this to yourself:

"Fibro Girl To The Recue!"

Remember this quote and take action to always get and use your antidotes on a daily basis for the rest of your life, to have less pain, more energy, and a happier and better quality of life:

"Feeling good is the antidote to feeling bad. Feeling pleasure is the antidote to feeling pain. Feeling happy

> **is the antidote to feeling sad. Feeling safe; loved and having faith, is the antidote to feeling fear."**

And don't forget to write a happy list of 10 things that make you happy, and incorporate as many of these into your life as possible on a daily basis. Along with your 10 most powerful positive music tracks, to keep you energised and feeling great, every day of your life!

ABOUT THE AUTHOR AND QUIRKY BOOKS

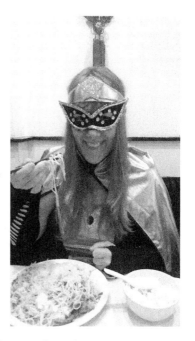

Author Sandra Bellamy, aka ACE Fibro Girl, was diagnosed with fibromyalgia in 2012 but does not let that stop her from living a full and active life to the max! Fibro Girl to the rescue! She lives in Exeter, in the UK, not far from the picturesque Quayside.

Sandra is the owner and founder of Quirky Books publishing company, a previously published Author and an award-winning businesswoman. She specialises in writing non-fiction.

A self-confessed night owl, Sandra prefers to write during the evening and night, as this is when she feels most focused and at her writing best. Sandra prides herself on being quirky, so if you are looking for books with a genre twist or out-of-the-box thinking, you will certainly love what Sandra and <u>Quirky Books</u> has to offer.

Non-fiction Quirky Books are specialist books for specific niches, and books that solve a problem with a difference or quirky twist. Quirky Books often defy traditional writing conventions in some way, and are first for crossing certain genres.

A NOTE FROM THE AUTHOR

Hey there, thanks so much for buying this book, I hope you got tons of value from it and will share it with all your fibro friends and those wanting to know more, and if you enjoyed it, please leave an honest review on Amazon.

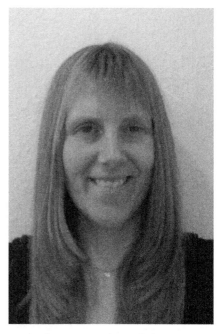

MY QUIRKY BOOKS MISSION:

My mission is to get YOU to EMBRACE YOUR QUIRKY in your life and business, to live a HAPPY, SUCCESSFUL, and FULFILLING existence! My aim is to empower you to live your best life through the written word, so you can be your true authentic self and the best version of you, regardless of what anyone else says, thinks, or does.

Many of us lack certain skills that would improve our quality of life, our communication skills, solve a problem, and take us to a more intelligent and knowledgeable level. That's where I come in. I have been training in the personal and professional development arena since 2012, the same year as my fibro diagnosis, with some of the top entrepreneurs and specialists in their field. My first event that year, along with coming to terms with my fibro diagnosis and taking charge of it, was truly life changing. It was the year I saw Tony Robbins for the first time live on stage and he got us to jump up and down to music, and talked about changing our state to change our mood and our life. He got us to hug strangers and up until that point I could never do this, and this was the start of my self-love journey and of opening up to others and leading a happy life. Prior to that year, I had depression for years, and I did not like my life and thought about death and dying fairly regularly and what's the point to life. But when I started to take responsibility of my fibro life and realised from going to that seminar, about all the skills, talents and experience I have to offer the world, it made me like myself and feel great about me, and now I love life and want to live forever.

I truly believe that writing is so powerful, you can literally change lives and the world through the written word and that to not pass on my valuable skills, knowledge and experience, in many aspects of life, would be a tragedy.

There is a wealth of knowledge available on the Internet, but it can still take considerable time to trundle through all the blog posts, videos and articles on a certain topic, and then it can get confusing as to which one is right, which one you should do, not to mention all of the distractions surrounding those. What you need is focus, and to have a book that gets to the heart of your problem, and gives you the answer you are looking for, in the quickest time, with minimal distraction, I hope you agree, this book does exactly that. If you need a problem solving and it's a topic I know about, your problem is solved, right here, with a book from Quirky Books, with more to come.

Find, follow, and connect with me at:

www.facebook.com/acefibrogirl
www.twitter.com/acefibrogirl
www.acefibrogirl.com

www.facebook.com/quirkybooksnet
www.facebook.com/sandrabellamyUK

www.twitter.com/quirkybooksnet
www.twitter.com/sandrabellamyUK

www.sandrabellamy.com
www.quirkybooks.net
www.quirkybooks.wordpress.com

SANDRA'S OTHER QUIRKY BOOKS TITLES TO READ THAT COMPLIMENT THIS BOOK

<u>ASEXUAL PERSPECTIVES: 47 ASEXUAL STORIES: LOVE, LIFE and SEX, ACElebration of ASEXUAL DIVERSITY</u>

<u>www.asexualise.com</u>

<u>www.asexualiseacademy.com</u>

<u>www.facebook.com/acexualise</u>

<u>www.facebook.com/acexualisedating</u>

<u>www.facebook.com/acexualiseacademy</u>

<u>www.twitter.com/asexualise</u>

Buy this book on Amazon or from my own digital store at <u>www.sellfy.com/quirkybooks.net</u>

You can also order the paperback edition from all good bookshops, under Author Sandra Bellamy, Publisher Quirky Books.

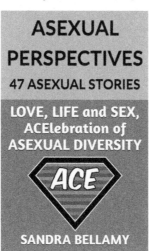

BREAK THROUGH THE BARRIERS OF REDUNDANCY TO GET BACK INTO WORK -AN A-Z 'HOW TO' GUIDE

www.beatredundancyblues.wordpress.com

www.facebook.com/beatredundancyblues

www.twitter.com/beatredundancyb

Shop for this book on Amazon and my own digital store at www.sellfy.com/quirkybooks.net

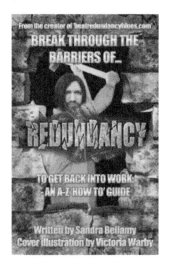

FURTHER READING AND RESOURCES

Other books you may want to check out:

Daniel Freeman and Jason Freeman, How To Keep Calm and Carry On, (Pearson, 2013).

Dr Frances Goodhart and Lucy Atkins, How To Feel Better, Practical ways to recover well from illness and injury, (Piatkus, 2013).

Brendon Burchard, The Motivation Manifesto, 9 Declarations to Claim Your Personal Power, (Hay House, 2014)

Brendon Burchard, The Charge, Activating The 10 Human Drives That Make You Feel Alive, (Free Press. A Division of Simon & Schuster, 2012).

Mark Rhodes, Think Your Way to Success, How to Develop a Winning Mindset and Achieve Amazing Results, (Capstone Publishing, 2012).

Elisabeth Wilson, Relax, 52 brilliant ideas to chill out, (Infinite Ideas, 2006).

If you want to know more about fibromyalgia:

National Fibromyalgia Association www.fmaware.org

National Fibromyalgia & Chronic Pain Association (NFMCPA) www.fmcpaware.org

Fibromyalgia Action UK www.fmauk.org

UK Fibromyalgia http://ukfibromyalgia.com

Facebook Groups:

Fibromyalgia Support Worldwide
https://www.facebook.com/groups/1412079755524155/

Fibro ABC's
https://www.facebook.com/groups/390415787696985/

Fibromyalgia & Invisible Illness Support Group
https://www.facebook.com/groups/fibrowarriorsfitandfab/

Printed in Great Britain
by Amazon